# A Whole-Body Approach
# to Slowing Down Aging

# A Whole-Body Approach to Slowing Down Aging

## Helping You Live Healthier and Longer

How to reduce the risks of cardiovascular
disease, osteoporosis, age-related cancer,
and loss of cognitive ability

Liang-Che Tao, MD, FCAP, FRCPC
Professor Emeritus of Pathology and Radiology
Indiana University School of Medicine
Indianapolis, Indiana

iUniverse, Inc.
Bloomington

# A Whole-Body Approach to Slowing Down Aging

## Helping You Live Healthier and Longer

*iUniverse books may be ordered through booksellers or by contacting:*
*iUniverse*
*1663 Liberty Drive*
*Bloomington, IN 47403*
*www.iuniverse.com*
*1-800-Authors (1-800-288-4677)*

*ISBN: 978-1-4502-9949-7 (pbk)*
*ISBN: 978-1-4502-9951-0 (ebk)*
*ISBN: 978-1-4502-9950-3 (hbk)*

*Library of Congress Control Number: 2011904979*

*Printed in the United States of America*
*iUniverse rev. date: 4/8/11*

This book is dedicated to seniors everywhere who wish to reduce the risks of cardiovascular disease, osteoporosis, age-related cancer, and loss of cognitive ability

# Contents

# Preface

Early in the twenty-first century, there is a proliferation of articles, books, and news reports on aging. Many health programs on this topic also crowd the television airwaves. This information overload seems to bombard us with conflicting schools of thought and many seemingly unconfirmed conclusions. Many opinions are simply based on the authors' own fields of knowledge and experience. And yet aging is a very complicated process. The complexities of getting older make it difficult to pinpoint why one person ages well while another looks and acts older than his age. At least five fields of in-depth knowledge are involved in revealing the long-sought secret of slowing down aging. These include biochemistry, physiology, pathology, nutrition, and clinical medicine. Discrepancies arise when research results are based not on a synthesis of these five fields but on splintered emphasis in one or two particular fields, without sufficient consideration of others.

I studied medicine twice. My first medical degree was from Peking University Health Science Center in 1954. I then practiced in Hong Kong for a few years. When I went to Alberta, Canada, in 1964, I was required to pass the medical licensing examination in order to practice medicine there. The qualifying examinations included basic medical sciences and clinical medicine. During the ten years after I graduated from Peking University, the basic medical sciences, especially biochemistry, had changed a great deal. I decided to repeat part of my medical studies and was admitted to the University of Alberta School of Medicine. When I studied biochemistry, physiology, and pathology for the second time, I appreciated those sciences in relation to human health much more than the first time. After I passed the medical licensing examination in Alberta, Canada, I decided to learn more about biochemistry, and I was accepted into the PhD program in biochemistry at the University of Alberta. In doing so, I stumbled upon a precious opportunity to learn advanced biochemistry, an up-and-coming field that consisted of protein biochemistry, lipid biochemistry, and nucleic acid biochemistry. Many years later, the knowledge I acquired during that time turned out to be very useful in assessing the reliability of various publications and presentations on the topic of aging.

After completing my residency training in pathology at the Toronto General Hospital and University of Toronto School of Medicine in Ontario, Canada, I gained a deeper appreciation about the body's natural defenses against diseases and its self-healing power. I wondered, *Why can't we take advantage of the body's natural protection during our senior years to prevent age-related diseases by bringing our bodies back to optimal physiological condition, including a fully functioning immune system?* Gradually, I formed my own views about an approach to slowing down the aging process.

In the 1990s, I was appointed professor of pathology, professor of radiology, and director of the cytopathology division at the Indiana University School of Medicine, in Indianapolis, Indiana. Due to a heavy workload and the pressures of directing a diagnostic clinic in the cancer center and the cytopathology division, as well as an improper lifestyle and poor eating habits, I was afflicted by numerous health problems, including hypertension, insomnia, chronic fatigue, gout, frequent episodes of cold sores and large areas of itchy rashes, constipation, severe hemorrhoids, anemia, and an old myocardial infarction (I still have an old scar in the anterior wall of my left ventricle).

After my retirement in 1999, I was relieved to not have to continue reading current professional journals in my own field, so I started to read publications on aging instead. During my retirement years, I have read over seventy aging-related books and more than one thousand research articles in the field. At the same time, I used myself as a guinea pig, trying to improve my health and slow down aging through natural and nutritional means, according to the theory that I was gradually forming. In so doing, I developed insights based on a synthesis of five fields (biochemistry, physiology, pathology, nutrition, and clinical medicine) regarding the process of aging and how to help the body regain control over its sovereign territory. Ten years later, now in my ninth decade of life, the numerous health problems I mentioned have practically disappeared. I have now put my thoughts together. This book explains my thesis and is a summary of my theory and ten years' work on aging.

In this book, I discuss a practical approach using natural and nutritional means to slow down the aging process based on published literature and my own experience. Although aging is inevitable, some systems that I will discuss have proven to help some people slow down—and possibly even reverse to a degree—a few of the aging processes. My work regarding improving health and slowing down aging offered much greater benefits than I ever imagined, and I believe that it will be helpful information available for those who may wish to use it. In this whole-body approach, the entire body works together synergistically to keep you healthier and living longer, helping you reduce the risks of cardiovascular disease, osteoporosis, age-related cancer, and loss of cognitive ability, which we used to assume were inescapable results of aging.

My experience in transforming my health through natural and nutritional means has convinced me that disease is not an inevitable part of aging. Preventive medicine requires a multifaceted approach: proper diet with necessary supplements, regular physical and mental exercises, and changes in improper lifestyle habits. All these measures will gradually bring your body back to optimal physiological condition, with a fully functioning immune system that will put you back on the road to better health.

# Chapter 1
# Primary Causes of Aging

We all have a chronological age, which is time-related and involves the celebration of birthdays, and our physiological age, which reflects the rate at which we are getting older. Everyone ages at the same chronological rate, but people do not age at the same physiological rates. The rates of aging throughout the body systems vary considerably from person to person.

Aging is universal, but each of us experiences it in different ways. We are the sum of our life experiences, and the condition of the various environments throughout our life affects our health, which, in turn, affects the aging process. Aging is influenced by many factors, including genetic makeup, lifestyle, eating habits, and environmental exposure. Therefore, our calendar age has little bearing on our real, physiological age.

Scientists have begun to recognize that misplaced, unnecessary, and prolonged inflammatory response may be the common root of many chronic degenerative diseases among seniors. Every disease I studied shared a common theme: inflammation was present. Whenever I look at a disease, everything from arthritis to heart disease, under a microscope, inflammation is always a component. Whether inflammation is simply a secondary response by the immune system or the key to the whole process of disease remains to be solved.

Genes are considered to be powerful predictors of health, susceptibility to diseases, and longevity. However, there is no question that healthy eating habits and a proper lifestyle are also powerful weapons against the susceptible genes we may be born with. Healthy living may delay many of the body changes that aging will bring. As long as no structural damage to a vital organ has occurred, it is never too late to start on the road to better health.

Primary causes of aging are summarized as follows:

## 1. Suboptimal Physiological Condition of the Body

For many of us, especially seniors, our bodies are no longer in optimal physiological condition due to improper lifestyle and eating habits and our increasingly toxic environment. Intracellular and extracellular tissue fluids outside of blood vessels, where most physiological functions take place, tend to gradually become acidic. The pH of the "body fluids" is traditionally believed to consistently be 7.4. In older literature, the term *body fluids* literally includes all the various kinds of fluids in the body, but in fact, this number refers primarily to the pH of the blood, which can fluctuate only slightly, from 7.35 to 7.45, due to the powerful, built-in homeostatic control mechanism by chemical buffer systems (including $H_2CO_3$ and $NaHCO_3$ systems, $Na_2HPO_4$ and $NaH_2PO_4$ systems, and the hemoglobin in the red blood cells). This homeostatic control mechanism in the circulating blood is extremely important; because the body cannot function properly if the pH of the blood falls below 7.35 or rises above 7.45.

When we examine sections of human tissues under a microscope with the help of special staining technique, we are able to observe a vast amount of non-circulating intracellular and extracellular tissue fluids in the space outside of blood vessels. These chemical buffer systems, which are so effective and vigilant in the circulating blood, do not work as efficiently in these relatively stationary tissue fluids. As a result, the pH of these intracellular and extracellular tissue fluids can fluctuate a lot more, depending on our body's alkaline reserve, which is affected by the foods we eat and the lifestyle we lead.

There appears to be much confusion about what constitutes "body fluids" in the older literature, due to lack of techniques to obtain more precise measurements of the amount of fluids in specific parts of the body. Now using bioelectrical impedance analysis (BIA), we are able to accurately measure that the total amount of body fluids in a man weighing 70 kg is approximately 40 L—57 percent of the body weight. In an infant, the total amount of body fluids is around 75 percent of the body weight, but it gradually decreases from birth to old age, with most of the decrease occurring during the first ten years of life. Obesity decreases the percentage of body fluids in the body to as low as 45 percent. The total amount of body fluids in a man weighing 70 kg can be broken down into three major compartments:

(1) **Intracellular tissue** fluid amounts to 62.5 percent, or 25 L. It represents a conglomeration of fluids from all the different cells. It is not homogeneous and does not circulate.

(2) **Extracellular tissue** (or interstitial) fluid amounts to 30 percent, or 12 L. It surrounds all the various cells in the space outside of blood vessels and does not circulate.

(3) **Plasma** amounts to 7.5 percent, or 3 L. It is the fluid portion of the blood inside blood vessels and circulates continuously throughout our lives.

The amount of plasma (blood) inside of blood vessels only accounts for 7.5 percent of the total amount of the body fluids. Circulating blood supplies nutrients and oxygen to the body's cells and transports waste products away from these cells to keep us alive; however, the majority of physiological functions take place via enzymatic reactions in the intracellular and extracellular tissue fluids. Thus, the pH of tissue fluids, which greatly affects the efficiency of enzymatic reactions, plays an important role in maintaining one's health. Restoring acid-alkaline balance in the tissue fluids to pH 7.4 is therefore key to maintaining good health.

Restoring the acid-alkaline balance in tissue fluids to a slightly alkaline condition (pH 7.4) allows optimal physiological functions, including metabolism, tissue repair, enzymatic reactions, and immune function. Lipofuscin, a granular, orange cellular waste product, is a substance that tends to build up in aging tissues. When we look at human tissues from seniors under a microscope, lipofuscin is frequently found in liver cells, heart muscle cells, and nerve cells. If the physiological condition of our body is suboptimal, lipofuscin accumulates over time and continuously builds up, binding fat and proteins together in the cells and interfering first with cell function, then tissue function, and then organ function. However, if the body's physiological condition improves, lipofuscin buildup decreases. Researchers found a significant decrease in lipofuscin buildup following supplementation with health-promoting resveratrol.

Many major studies (including a long-range study by the European Prospective Investigation into Cancer and Nutrition that monitored 470,000 people in ten different countries, and another study by the Department of Epidemiology at Harvard University following 91,000 nurses over twelve years) found that increased risks of colon, breast, and prostate cancer were closely linked to long-standing, high consumption of red meat, refined sugar, and/or refined grains, all of which are acidifying foods. They also found that reduced red meat consumption was associated with decreased risk of colon cancer (*Journal of the National Cancer Institute*, No. 12, 2005). All these studies appear to say that high and prolonged consumption of acidifying foods increases the acidity in the tissue fluids (even though the pH of the blood remains 7.4), resulting in the development of cancer. I will discuss this further in chapter 8.

In recent years, medical doctors have been trying to make use of the adjustment of acid-alkaline balance in the tissue fluids to correct health problems. One recent study in the *Journal of Clinical Endocrinology and Metabolism*, January 2009, by Dr. Dawson-Hughes and his colleagues is such an example. In this study, 171 healthy men and women aged fifty and older were treated with either alkaline bicarbonate or no bicarbonate. Those receiving alkaline bicarbonate, in an amount equivalent to nine servings of fruits and vegetables daily, experienced much lower levels of calcium loss in the urine, as well as a loss of N-telopeptide, the biochemical marker of bone resorption. Dr. Dawson-Hughes's team concluded that increasing the alkaline content of the diet by eating more fruits and vegetables can be used as a safe and low-cost approach to preventing osteoporosis and improving bone health in older Americans. You can discover more about this finding in chapter 7.

The natural protection against diseases and self-healing power of the human body is powerful only if the body is in optimal physiological condition, with a healthy pH of 7.4 in the tissue fluids. As a result of improper lifestyle, eating habits, and environmental changes, the tissue fluids gradually become acidic. Bacteria are often found in aging arthritic joints, arterial plaques, gums, tooth cavities, tonsils, and intestinal tracts. In fact, the mouth is the habitat of many bacteria, and there are as much as 500 million bacteria per milliliter of saliva. The presence of bacterial products, including organic acids, amines, and thiols, causes saliva to sometimes carry a foul odor. Numerous microbial species may infest us. Populations of bacteria and fungi may thrive throughout the body without causing acute disease, yet they produce copious acid waste products. Furthermore, the human body makes acid as a natural by-product of metabolism, but it produces nothing alkaline. These factors, if they are not corrected, all contribute to the rise of acidic levels in the tissue fluids.

The proper function of the various organs is mostly carried out by enzymatic reactions that continually take place in the intracellular and extracellular tissue fluids of our body. All enzymes have an optimum pH range and can only perform their tasks correctly and efficiently in an environment with a clearly defined pH; otherwise their activity can be disrupted and even cease completely. When enzymatic activity is merely slowed down, illness appears. Following a long period of acidic tissue fluids, various physiological functions of the body, including immune function, deteriorate. The acidification of the internal terrain of our body is in fact the source of many health troubles.

## 2. Weakened Immune System

The human immune system, which protects our body from internal or foreign invaders, may not function properly if our body suffers from multiple nutritional deficiencies or suppression of the central nervous system due to stress, worries, and/or pressure. In order to function optimally, the immune system needs vitamins, essential minerals, essential amino acids, and essential fatty acids. People whose diets are low in certain nutrients, notably the minerals iron, selenium, magnesium, calcium, and zinc, and the vitamins A, B, C, and D, tend to have fewer and less active natural killer (NK) cells, a group of white blood cells that are the body's vital first line of defense against disease. Vitamin E maintains an adequate arsenal of T lymphocytes, virus-fighting immune cells that typically decline with age. Research also shows that vitamin D is extremely important for the immune system. It helps regulate T lymphocytes and turns on the gene that produces cathelicidin, a natural antimicrobial chemical compound that fights infection (*Future Microbiology*, November 2009).

Essential amino acids, such as lysine, tryptophan, etc., are also necessary for healthy cellular growth and immunity. However, they cannot be produced by our bodies. The sources of essential omega-3 fatty acids, which are important components for cell membrane formation, nerve-impulse conduction, hormone production, metabolic function, brain function, and immune function, are becoming less available through food sources found in supermarkets. Omega-3 fatty acid molecules are a biochemical by-product of the happy meeting of sunlight and carbon dioxide in the chloroplasts of terrestrial plants and marine algae. The production of omega-3 fatty acids in nature has been gradually decreased by human intervention. For example, cattle are no longer grass-fed; chickens are raised in cages and stuffed full of corn; and farm-raised salmon, trout, and steelheads are fed soy pallets.

Furthermore, chronic mental stress, whether it stems from external pressure or internal perception, also impairs immunity. People who experience higher levels of stress or negative moods are more susceptible to infection, develop more severe illnesses, and take longer to heal.

In addition to mental stress, physical stress can be caused by trauma and wounds. Both mental and physical stresses can trigger the production of cortisol, a hormone that can have dire consequences for your health. When a high level of cortisol circulates in the body for long periods of time, it will raise blood glucose, elevate blood pressure, decalcify bones, destroy brain cells, and eventually damage the immune system.

Chronic alcohol abuse and smoking can also suppress immune system. Alcohol impedes the ability of white blood cells to travel to infected sites, gobble up and destroy foreign invaders, and identify dysplastic cells and malignant cells. As a result, alcoholics are more susceptible to bacterial diseases and have an increased risk of developing cancer.

### 3. Increased Free radical Attacks

In the 1950s, Denham Harman, professor emeritus of medicine at the University of Nebraska, identified free radicals as atoms or molecules that are missing one of their two electrons. They are unstable and will try to take another electron from any other atom or molecule in the immediate environment. If a free radical acquires an electron from the atom or molecule next to it, then that atom or molecule may become a free radical. In turn, the new free radical attacks an atom or molecule next to it, and so on, creating a chain reaction of atoms or molecules that are desperately seeking an electron. Dr. Harman postulated that it is the damage to these molecules that leads to aging. The medical community ignored Harman's theory for some twenty years. Scientists finally found evidence of the free radical theory in the biological aging process, and it began to gain acceptance.

As mitochondria (microscopic bodies in cells containing enzymes responsible for energy production) convert nutrients into energy, they generate corrosive free radicals. Free radicals are also produced as part of many other enzymatic reactions that our body performs to sustain life. In addition, free radicals are created in very high levels throughout the body whenever there is trauma, infection, or inflammation.

Free radicals are really by-products of metabolism and act like highly reactive oxygen molecules. Every cell in our body receives an estimated 10,000 free radical hits daily. By reacting with nearby fats, proteins, and nucleic acids, free radicals give rise to many diseases. Those intracellular free radicals can attack DNA and cause cell death or mutations, resulting in precancerous dysplastic cells. Extracellular free radicals foster everything from cataracts, arthritis, and cardiovascular disease to loss of cognitive ability. In heart disease, free radicals promote the oxidation of low-density lipoprotein (LDL) cholesterol, which tends to accumulate as fatty plaques in the artery walls and may further clog or obstruct the arteries. The brain, which consists of 60 percent of fats with elevated levels of polyunsaturated fatty acids, the targets of lipid peroxidation, is uniquely vulnerable to oxidative injuries from increased free radical attacks. In nerve cells, free radical attacks dramatically cut back on the nerve cells' ability to communicate, leading to age-related cognitive decline (see chapter 9).

However, the healthy body, especially in young people, produces a profusion of superoxide dismutase (SOD), a powerful free radical killer that mops up free radicals. SODs are present in almost all cells and in extracellular tissue fluids. In seniors, the production of SOD is greatly reduced, and free radical attacks may thus become out of control. Although cells repair more than 99 percent of the ensuing damage, mistakes add up. The accumulation of damage over the decades impairs cells, then tissues, then organs, and may eventually age the whole person.

When we are young and healthy, our bodies are equipped with a fully functioning immune system, capable of destroying foreign invaders, and strong self-healing powers. However, throughout years of improper lifestyle, unhealthy eating habits, and an increasingly toxic environment, many of us are bombarded by various adverse factors on a constant basis. Our bodies are no longer in optimal physiological condition. Our weakened immune system becomes vulnerable to the development of a host of chronic degenerative diseases. In addition to that, the production of protective, endogenous free radical killers is greatly reduced with age, permitting frequent free radical attacks. Dysfunction in one area is echoed in other areas. Aging affects not only isolated areas of the body but eventually the body as a whole.

# Chapter 2
# A Whole-Body Approach
# to Slowing Down Aging

In 1900, life expectancy in the United States was fifty years (*National Vital Statistics Reports*, Vol. 58, No. 21). During the past century, life expectancy has increased by nearly thirty years in the United States; this is clearly the result of the advancements made in medical science during the past fifty years and improvements in nutrition and sanitation. Health is not something that just happens, and there is much that we can do to slow down the aging process. The big questions of why we age and which experiences we can incorporate or change are coming into focus. There is no doubt that we can age better by eating healthfully, exercising regularly, avoiding alcohol and cigarettes, maintaining inner peace, and being mentally active. But can we realistically expect to further extend our life span?

Researchers have already accomplished some good results in animal experiments. One of these studies focuses on calorie restriction, which seems to preserve bone mass, immune function, brain function, and skin thickness. It appears that calorie restriction may slow the production of free radicals and thus help the body counter them more efficiently. Yet results related to the human body are still uncertain.

Another approach is to manipulate hormones, such as human growth hormones, thymus hormones, and sex hormones, but so far no research has conclusively shown that any of these hormones can alter life span.

All of these studies hold a fairly obvious lesson. Life itself is mortal, and our bodies are designed to last only so long. But with care and maintenance, they will live beyond their warranties.

In this chapter I will discuss a whole-body approach, in which the whole body works synergistically to protect your health and help you live longer. This whole-body approach is based on published literature and the insights that emerged during the ten years in which I tried to use natural and nutritional means to correct all kinds of health problems that I encountered. My results are very encouraging; this approach brought about a considerable improvement to my health. It even appears to have given me an edge on reversing the aging process. Once I worked out the primary causes of aging, I was able to design a course of therapeutic intervention.

### 1. Bring your body back to optimal physiological condition, with a healthy pH of 7.4 in the tissue fluids

When healthy, the pH of blood is 7.4; the pH of tissue fluids is 7.4; and the pH of fasting saliva is also 7.4. But in people with improper eating habits and lifestyle, as well as health problems, the pH of the tissue fluids may vary, though the pH of blood often remains 7.4. Since the pH of the blood can fluctuate only very slightly due to the powerful, built-in homeostatic control mechanism, testing it is not the best means to indicate the overall pH balance in our body.

As discussed in chapter 1, when we look at sections of human tissues under a microscope, we observe the presence of a vast amount of intracellular and extracellular tissue fluids in the space outside of blood vessels. In practice, however, there is no easy way to collect them for the purpose of pH testing. Properly collected fasting saliva may serve this purpose. The pH of fasting saliva offers a window through which we can assess the overall pH balance in our body, which, in turn, reflects our general physiological condition.

Saliva is produced in the salivary glands. It is composed of 98 percent water and 2 percent other compounds, such as electrolytes, mucus, and various enzymes. As part of the initial process of food digestion, the enzymes in the saliva break down some of the starch and fat in the foods. There are three types of major salivary glands, namely parotid, submandibular, and sublingual. There are two types of secretory cells in salivary glands, including serous and mucous.

In a healthy person, the parotid and submandibular glands produce approximately one liter of saliva per day. During sleep, the amount of saliva greatly decreases; most saliva is secreted by the sublingual gland to keep the mucosa of the mouth moist. The saliva stimulated by sympathetic innervation is thicker and contains digestive enzymes, which are produced by the serous cells in the submandibular and parotic glands. During sleep, the saliva stimulated by parasympathetic innervation is more watery and mostly produced in the sublingual glands.

While you eat, the digestive enzymes, including amylase, salivary lipase, and salivary lactoperoxidase, are produced by serous cells of the parotid and submandibular glands. All these digestive enzymes may affect a saliva pH reading. During sleep, most of the saliva is produced by the mucous cells of the sublingual gland, which do not produce digestive enzymes. Therefore, the pH of the watery saliva produced by the sublingual gland is most consistent with the pH of its surrounding tissue fluids and thus reflects your general physiological condition. The morning fasting saliva pH test offers a good chance to understand the pH of your tissue fluids.

You can use litmus paper (one that measures pH between 4.5 and 8.5 is good enough; it's available at laboratory suppliers and some supplement-manufacturing companies) to do the saliva pH test, but you need to wait at least three hours after eating or drinking, until the stomach is empty. If done too soon, the pH of the saliva may be affected by the digestive enzymes present in the saliva during eating, and the reading becomes inaccurate. This is the reason why some people get inconsistent results for saliva pH tests. According to my experience, the best time to do the saliva pH test is in the morning, just after you get out of bed, before you brush your teeth. This morning fasting saliva pH test can provide you rather accurate and consistent results.

Before you do the morning fasting saliva pH test, fill your mouth with saliva and then swallow it. Do this again and then a third time to ensure that the saliva is clean and contains no bacterial acid products. Put some saliva onto the litmus paper. Or use a spoon to hold the saliva, and dip the litmus paper in it. Shake off excess saliva, which may dilute the color. Wait about thirty seconds, and compare the color to the chart that comes with the litmus paper.

Most healthy young children have a pH of 7.4 for the morning fasting saliva pH test. More than half of adults over the age of sixty have an unhealthy pH of 6.4 or lower, and many cancer patients, especially when they are at the terminal stage, receive a pH reading of between 5.4 and 6.4 or lower. The pH scale goes from 0 to 14 and is logarithmic, which means that each step is ten times the previous. In other words, a pH of 5.4 is ten times more acidic than 6.4, and a hundred times more acidic than 7.4.

It takes a 1000 glasses of mineral water with a pH of 9.4 to bring the pH of a glass of strongly acidifying soft drink (containing phosphates) that has a pH of 2.4 up to a pH of 7.4. However, in the circulating blood of our bodies are powerful, built-in homeostatic control buffer systems, able to bring up the pH of a glass of strongly acidifying soft drink to pH 7.4 in no time once it is absorbed. In practice, a steady daily diet of three or four cans of strongly acidifying soft drinks over a long period of time (say, years) will certainly drain the alkaline reserve in the body and thus tilt the pH of tissue fluids (not blood) toward acidity.

Before I started my own anti-aging program, the pH of my morning fasting saliva was an unhealthy 6.4. (In retrospect, that was obviously due to excess consumption of strongly acidifying soft drinks and red meat.) It took me more than a year to bring the pH from the unhealthy 6.4 up to a stabilized, healthy pH of between 7.2 and 7.6 for the morning fasting saliva pH test. Let me discuss the ways to raise the alkalinity in tissue fluids through diet.

A.  Eat more alkalizing foods

The "rule of thumb" is to eat 20 percent acidifying foods and 80 percent alkalizing foods. When the pH readings of your morning fasting saliva pH tests appear healthy and stabilized, between pH 7.2 and 7.6, you can adjust the rule and increase acidifying foods to 30 percent if you wish. In practice, it's not easy to measure the ratio of the amounts of different kinds of foods. You can use the pH reading of the morning fasting saliva pH tests as a guide to make adjustments to the various portions of acidifying and alkalizing foods.

The acidifying or alkalizing degree of foods largely depends on the products after digestion. For instance, after digestion, beef contains sulfuric, phosphoric, and uric acids plus amino acids and is, therefore, an acidifying food. Lemon and vinegar, although acidic in taste, after digestion are actually alkalizing. White bread and refined sugar are not at all acidic to the taste, but they are acidifying foods.

In the literature, some authors determine the nature of a food by burning the food and then mixing the ash with water. Whether the solution is acidic or alkaline, the food is then labeled as acidic or alkaline. However, because this method of determining the nature of food is not based on the products after digestion, this approach can be quite misleading.

Products that are strongly acidic after digestion come primarily from animal proteins. Vegetables and fruits are predominantly metabolized to alkaline bicarbonate. Generally speaking, red meat, poultry, and fish are acidifying foods. Milk and other dairy foods are slightly acidifying. All grains and nuts are also acidifying. Cheese and egg yolk are strongly acidifying, while egg white is slightly acidifying. Most fruits and berries except persimmon are alkalizing. Most vegetables, melons, and peas are also alkalizing.

B.  Drink slightly alkaline water and alkalizing beverages

Most people do not realize that the water or beverages you drink every day also contribute to the pH level of tissue fluids. This usually happens when you drink from the same source of water or drink the same kind of beverages for a prolonged period of time (say, for years). In the past, we only emphasized safe drinking water, meaning the water we drink should be free of bacteria, parasitic cysts, toxic chemicals and some heavy metals. Now we should also emphasize the importance of healthy drinking water: water that has a pH close to 7.4 and contains some essential minerals that our body needs.

If you want to test the tap water in your home, boil it first to get rid of chlorine present in the water, which will tilt the pH toward acidity. In fact, the pH of tap water in most cities in this country is higher than that of most bottled drinking water, which is usually based on municipal water treated with reverse osmosis and some additives. Boil tap water before you drink it.

Out of curiosity, I tested all the bottled drinking water sold in the supermarkets. To my surprise, most of them, except natural mineral and spring waters, were between pH 6.2 and 6.6. Even the one called Alpine Spring Water, with a picture showing mountains covered with snow, was tested at pH 6.4. According to my tests, all natural mineral and spring waters tested alkaline.

When water contains more acidic than alkaline minerals, it is said to be acidic. Acidic minerals are sulfur, chlorine, phosphorus, fluoride, iodine, and silicon. Alkaline minerals include calcium, sodium, potassium, magnesium, cobalt, and copper. The acidifying or alkalizing degree of drinking water largely depends on the balance of acidic and alkaline minerals present in the water, which, unlike in foods, are already at the appropriate molecular level to be absorbed by the intestinal tract.

Water filtered by a reverse osmosis system was claimed to be the best drinking water, and I have a reverse osmosis system installed in my home. It tested at pH 6.0! This unacceptable pH level occurs simply because alkaline minerals are removed during membrane filtration. It is safe drinking water but not suitable for drinking for a prolonged period of time. Water treated by a water softener system contains too much sodium and is also not suitable for long-term drinking.

At the present time, most bottled drinking water sold in some Asian countries, including Japan, South Korea, and China, indicates the pH of the water on the bottle label, but not in North America.

Beverages like fruit juices, teas, and coffee (without added sugar and cream) are generally alkalizing; however, most carbonated beverages are acidifying, and those containing phosphates and a large amount of sugar are even strongly acidifying, with pH readings between 2.0 and 2.5.

C. Participate in physical exercise

The benefits of regular exercise to the cardiovascular and immune systems are well documented in many articles and books. Dr. David Dunstan, an Australian researcher, recently reported his study in *Circulation: Journal of the American Heart Association*. He and his coworkers tracked 8,800 people for an average of six years and found that those who watched TV for more than four hours a day were 46 percent more likely to die of any cause and 80 percent more likely to die of cardiovascular disease than people spending less than two hours a day in front of the TV. Research also showed the important role of muscle movement in how the body processed blood sugar and blood fats. The absence of movement can slow down our metabolic processes. After just a few hours of inactivity, an enzyme called lipoprotein lipase that pulls fat from the blood shut down. Instead of fat being transported to muscle tissue where it was burned as fuel, fat accumulated in the bloodstream, where over time it promoted atherosclerosis of the artery walls, leading to cardiovascular disease (*Circulation*, January 2010).

I would like to point out that regular exercise also helps contribute to the ideal level of tissue fluid pH. By increasing the excretion of acidic waste through perspiration (sweat) and by increasing carbon dioxide output through expiration, exercise can tilt the pH of tissue fluids toward alkalinity.

## 2. Boost the immune system

Our bodies are under constant attack from bacteria and viruses. A healthy immune system, well armed with natural killer (NK) cells, T and B lymphocytes, leucocytes, plasma cells, macrophages, antibodies, and other substances, can destroy or inactivate those invaders and can also eliminate precancerous dysplastic cells from within our body.

One key result of the activation of the immune system is the inflammatory response. Inflammation must stay where it is supposed to stay and end when it is supposed to end. The inflammatory response is tightly regulated by the immune system in coordination with certain hormones. The weakened immune system may fail to regulate the inflammatory response, leading to health troubles. If inflammation is too little and too late, bacteria or viruses can get the upper hand; on the other hand, if it is too much and too long or occurs when it is unnecessary, other health problems result.

Fortunately, there are steps we can take to boost our immune system, including proper diet, taking supplements wisely, regular exercise, relieving stress, and practicing other healthy behaviors. These measures offer protection even in seniors, challenging the long held notion that immunity inevitably declines with age. Here's what you can do to enhance your immune system.

A.  Proper diet with necessary supplements

In order to guarantee peak performance of the immune system, the body needs to have sufficient amounts of vitamins A, B, C, D, E, and K (thirteen kinds altogether); various essential minerals and trace elements, such as iron, selenium, calcium, and zinc (sixteen kinds), eight essential amino acids, such as lysine, tryptophan, etc., and two essential fatty acids, including omega-3 (alpha-linolenic acid) and omega-6 (linoleic acid).

In theory, a healthful diet should provide a sufficient amount of the nutrients the body needs. However, only when foods are fully digested down to the molecular level are these nutrients absorbed and put to use. In practice, chronic gastrointestinal disorders and pancreatitis impair digestion and abso rption. Resection of a gallbladder undermines absorption of lipid nutrients. Other people who may also need supplements to plug the nutritional gaps include dieters, picky eaters, strict vegetarians, pregnant women, and seniors.

Furthermore, the sources of some important nutrients, such as omega-3 fatty acids, have become fewer, because, as I have mentioned, farm-raised cattle are no longer grass-fed, chickens are raised in cages and fed with corn, and salmon, trout, and steelheads are commonly farm-raised and fed with soy pallets. In addition, most fish is contaminated with mercury and polychlorinated biphenyls (PCBs). According to federal health warnings analyzed by the Environmental Working Group, fish from more than 1,660 US waterways are so contaminated with mercury that they should not be eaten, or eaten only in limited amounts.

Soil can be depleted of certain minerals, such as boron and selenium, by intensive farming and excessive use of soluble chemical fertilizers; vegetables subsequently grown in those areas have relatively low nutritional content. Levels of boron, which is an important trace element for the human body, have dropped considerably in the last fifty years in this country (*Journal of the American Dietetic Association*, May 1991). This is part of the reason why we can no longer depend on food sources for adequate nutritional needs. Supplementation with vitamins and minerals has become necessary to keep you healthy (see chapter 3).

In the process of aging, it appears that what we eat plays an important role in our health. In Japan sixty years ago, Okinawans once boasted the longest life expectancy in the world. But the postwar American administration, which didn't end until 1972, introduced and popularized the standard American diet. Many residents, whose diet was originally high in marine omega-3 fatty acids and foods of plant origins, switched to an American diet rich in red meat, saturated fat, and seed-based, omega-6 vegetable oils. Consequently, their reign as the champions of longevity also ended. By 1990, life expectancy among Okinawan males had plunged to fifth among all regions of Japan. They also experienced a rise in cancer, cardiovascular disease, and diabetes. In 1990, the death rates for Okinawan males under age fifty were the highest of any place in Japan (Carper, J., *Your Miracle Brain*. Harper, 2000).

As a matter of fact, fats are as crucial to a healthy body as protein is. The brain itself is 60 percent fat. The key to good health lies in eating the best possible fats sufficient for our body's need. Those beneficial fats are marine omega-3 fatty acids, which are essential for healthy growth, metabolism, oxygen transfer, brain and nerve tissue function, and immune function. However, the human body cannot manufacture them.

There are two specific forms of omega-3s: docosahexaenoic acid (DHA) and eicosapentaenoic acid (EPA). DHA has a cylindrical shape and can compress and twist, switching between hundreds of different shapes thousands of times a second. The molecule is particularly abundant in the wings of hummingbirds, the tails of rattlesnakes, the tails of sperm, the rods and cones of the retinas, and neurons. DHA is the main structural fatty acid in the gray matter of the brain and retina of the eye. It is essential for brain and eye function. A neuron that is high in DHA molecules is virtually liquid, allowing for more effective reception of serotonin, dopamine, and other neurotransmitters (see chapter 9). EPA omega-3 fatty acids are also beneficial to health. They can reduce blood clotting and restrain the inflammatory response in tissues.

Marine omega-3 fatty acids are long-chain molecules (which refers to the number of carbon atoms in the omega-3 molecules) and contain high levels of already synthesized DHA and EPA that are ready for use by cells. Plant-derived omega-3s found in olive oil, flaxseed oil, avocado, canola oil, and walnut are short-chain molecules that have to be converted to long-chain omega-3s before the human body can fully make use of them.

Long-chain omega-3s, found in marine fishes and other seafood, are the only kind of polyunsaturated fatty acids proven to exert maximum health benefits to our body. Short-chain, plant-derived omega-3s cannot be further synthesized to DHA and EPA by plants and therefore cannot replace long-chain omega-3 fatty acids. Although our body can convert them to long-chain omega-3s, the amounts produced are limited. The body converts no more than 10 percent of short-chain, plant-derived omega-3s to usable long-chain omega-3s, and they are mainly EPA and very little DHA. Although plant-derived omega-3 fatty acids are also beneficial to health, they are relatively poor sources of DHA.

Increasingly, omega-6 fatty acids are present in larger amounts in our diet. Conversely, an adequate supply of long-chain omega-3 fatty acids seems to be much more difficult to obtain. The ratio of omega-6 to omega-3 fatty acids obtained through the average American diet has become more like 20:1, while the ideal healthy ratio is 2:1. This imbalance may produce negative repercussions *vis-à-vis* the development of cardiovascular disease, certain age-related cancers, and loss of cognitive ability, because excess omega-6s are used by the body to synthesize series 2 prostaglandins (PGE-2s), which suppress immune cells and play a role in extensive chronic inflammation. In contrast, anti-inflammatory EPA omega-3 fatty acids are scant in our average American diet.

Thus, adding good quality marine omega-3 fatty acid (fish oil) soft gels to a proper diet seems necessary for good health at the present time. Be careful—many supplements labeled as rich in omega-3s or fortified with omega-3s, without mentioning the source of omega-3s, are in fact the cheaper, plant-derived omega-3 fatty acids.

B.  Stress relief

Stress is as much of a risk factor for heart attacks and strokes as severe obesity and smoking. Stress has been linked to impaired immunity, worsening asthma, depression, chronic pain, and gastrointestinal problems. Cortisol, a stress hormone, is released by the adrenal glands when you are faced with a major stressor. It suppresses your immune system and decreases your ability to fight infection; it also makes you more susceptible to all kinds of diseases. Stress may also prompt unhealthy behaviors such as alcohol abuse, sleep deprivation, and smoking (Oz, M. C. and Roizen, M. F., *Staying Young*. Free Press 2007).

As a first step toward gaining control, consider what areas in your life provoke stress. Common sources of stress include job strain, raising children, a rushed daily schedule, and financial worries. Stress-reduction programs are strongly recommended. Individual stress management consultations or programs are offered by some hospitals and medical schools. Another option is to develop self-help strategies, such as aerobic exercise, yoga, and tai chi, and add some other forms of relaxation, such as hobbies, a massage, listening to music, and meditation.

### C. Don't compromise the immune system

As modern life becomes more sophisticated, the chance of toxic chemicals entering your body is also greatly increased. Environmental contamination by toxic chemicals that enter the food chain and our drinking water is now a reality. Every day we are bombarded with some chemical substances that can cause damage to our bodies at the cellular level. For instance, we live in homes that may harbor vinyl chloride, asbestos, lead-based paints, glue used in carpeting, and formaldehyde, found in plywood, paints, plastics, detergents, and particle board. We use insecticides to rid our homes of pests and herbicides to rid our lawns of weeds. Added to these potential dangers are preservatives and chemical additives in our foods, such as sodium nitrites in processed meats. During cooking, nitrites in meat react with degradation products of amino acids, forming nitrosamines, which are known carcinogens.

At the present time, many food containers are made of plastic. Not all plastic containers are made of the same material. Those marked on the bottom of each container within a triangle as 3, 6, and 7 are harmful to health, because such plastic food containers may release toxic substances from the plastic additives into the food. People are exposed to many chemical substances that may do harm even at low levels, such as phthalates (found in food containers, and nail polish), flame retardants (found in furniture, and electronics), and fluoropolymers (like Teflon in cookware and gears).

Bisphenol A (BPA) is found in a staggering array of products, from beer and food cans to all kinds of plastics, and is manufactured at the rate of 6 billion pounds a year. Aluminum cans are now coated with a plastic lining to prevent corrosion and protect the liquid contents from acquiring a metallic flavor. These plastic liners contain BPA. A recent analysis in *Consumer Reports* (December 2009) indicated that some juices and canned foods contain measurable amounts of BPA, and heating food containers labeled "microwave safe" causes high doses of BPA to leach into the food. BPA acts like the female hormone estrogen and blocks the male hormone androgen. In animal studies, it has been linked to prostate damage, lower sperm counts, and the possibility of cancer. Human studies link BPA to miscarriages, breast cancer in women, and male sexual dysfunction. A recent study in China reported that workers exposed to higher levels of BPA were found to have increased incidences of erectile dysfunction.

High temperature cooking and barbecuing meat may also generate carcinogens called *heterocyclic amines*.

At no other time in history has the human body been bombarded by so many adverse factors on a consistent basis. For the time being, the best you can do is to avoid these toxic chemicals as much as you can.

Furthermore, some medications that we are taking may also be potentially toxic to our body. The liver is the center of detoxification. The lining cells of liver sinusoids, called Kupffer cells (a kind of immune cell), are the first line of defense to fight off these toxic effects. However, prolonged use of such medications can deplete the Kupffer cells and cause damage to the liver cells, leading to liver failure. In the United States, acetaminophen-related liver problems occur in just a tiny fraction of the drug's users, but it still causes 450 deaths and 56,000 emergency room visits a year. The accumulation of toxic chemicals increases the toxic burden in our body. The immune system is then compromised or may even be destroyed (see chapter 4).

### 3. Control free radical attacks

This is especially important for seniors, because as we age, the production of superoxide dismutases (SODs) by the body is greatly decreased. When mitochondria in cells convert nutrients into energy, they generate numerous corrosive free radicals at the same time. There are hundreds of mitochondria per cell. Free radicals are also produced as part of many other enzymatic reactions that our body performs to sustain life. In addition, free radicals are created in very high levels throughout the body whenever there is trauma, infection, or inflammation. For instance, chronic cigarette smoking generates abundant free radicals because of accompanying chronic bronchitis, and chronic alcohol drinking also produces a high level of free radicals because of alcoholic hepatitis.

Every cell in our body receives an estimated 10,000 free radical hits daily, causing oxidative damage to our body. Free radicals, which act like highly reactive oxygen molecules, may react with the nucleic acid, proteins, and fats. Those intracellular free radicals can attack DNA and cause cell death or mutations that incite cells to aberrant behavior, resulting in precancerous dysplastic cells. In fact, 90 percent of us, especially seniors, carry precancerous dysplastic cells in various organs. However, if your immune system is in optimal condition, the immune cells will treat these dysplastic cells as foreign invaders and kill them before they progress into cancer cells. Those extracellular free radicals may react with nearby proteins and fats and promote cataracts, arthritis, cardiovascular disease, and even loss of cognitive ability.

Fortunately, these free radicals can be rendered harmless if we take proper antioxidants. Antioxidants are a chemical substance that can donate an electron to a free radical without contributing harm, thus putting an end to the destructive damage of cells and tissues.

The main antioxidants can be grouped into four categories:

(1) Vitamins, including A (and carotenoids), C, and E

(2) Minerals, including zinc, selenium, and manganese

(3) Chemicals, including alpha-lipoic acid, coenzyme Q10 (CoQ10), resveratrol, quercetin, L-carnitine, superoxide dismutase, and glutathione

(4) Hormones, including melatonin and DHEA

Wise use of antioxidants may help your body control free radical attacks (see chapter 5).

In short, there has never been a better time to grow old. Life expectancy shot up dramatically in the last century. Remember, in 1900, life expectancy was fifty in the United States. Today there are more fifty-year-olds than ever before in history, and they can anticipate another full thirty years, and maybe more. The challenge in this century is to find ways to curtail what we used to think of as the inevitable signs of aging, such as cardiovascular disease, osteoporosis, development of age-related cancers, and loss of cognitive ability, in order to maintain quality of life. Research has already shown that we have a lot of control over our own health in reducing the risks of these diseases.

The approaches to slowing down the aging process just discussed, including (1) bringing your body back to optimal physiological condition, (2) boosting your immune system, and (3) controlling free-radical attacks, are basically a whole-body approach. This approach to reducing risks for a host of chronic degenerative diseases among seniors is considered preventive, but it may also be therapeutic in people in whom no structural damage of a vital organ has occurred.

This whole-body approach is a departure from the current approach to health management, which tends to compartmentalize the human body into various organs and their corresponding diseases. However, aging is a systemic process that affects not simply an isolated organ of our body but the body as a whole. Dysfunction in one area is often echoed in other areas. This is the basic consideration for the whole-body approach. For instance, to reduce the risk of heart attacks in seniors, currently patients are given statin-type drugs to lower total blood cholesterol and LDL levels and raise HDL levels, plus aspirin or Plavix to prevent blood clot formation. Are these measures really enough to reduce the risk of heart attacks?

A clinical trial of Torcetrapib, a drug that can raise HDL and lower total cholesterol and LDL, was halted midstream because the drug seemed to cause heart attacks and strokes rather than prevent them. On December 2, 2006, Pfizer issued a press release stating that clinical trials and manufacturing of Torcetrapib were halted due to safety concerns.

In Israel, due to religious proscriptions that forbid consumption of meat and milk products in the same meal, butter is virtually excluded; cooking techniques rely heavily on margarine, as well as sunflower oil, which is rich in omega-6 fatty acids. As a result, Israelis, distinguished by one of the lowest cholesterol levels in Western countries, have one of the highest rates of cardiovascular disease. Elliot Berry, MD, at Hadassah University in Jerusalem, identified the link between cardiovascular disease and the high trans fat and omega-6 fatty acid levels in Israelis, which promotes inflammation, resulting in a rise in cardiovascular disease. Australian aborigines also have low cholesterol levels but high rates of heart disease.

On the other hand, Greenland's Inuit people get most of their calories from fish, seal blubber, and whale meat. In spite of their high cholesterol intake, they rarely die from heart disease. The Swiss have higher cholesterol levels than those of most Americans, but their rate of heart disease is lower. These findings and reports appear to indicate that there are some other contributing factors involved in the pathogenesis of heart attacks. After all, a high cholesterol level is just one of the risk factors for coronary heart disease.

Increased free radical attacks after high protein and high fat meals promote the oxidation of LDL, resulting in an increased accumulation of fatty plaques in the arterial walls; the corrosive homocysteine produced after digesting animal protein, especially in people with vitamin B-12 and folic acid deficiencies, can damage endothelial cells, which line artery walls, promoting atherosclerosis and blood clot formation. Nowadays, we tend to consume a great amount of processed foods, such as cookies, crackers, pastries, pizza, or potato chips, which contain trans fats, which are even more proinflammatory than excess omega-6s and also have a stronger adverse effect on artery walls than saturated fat. All these factors may play a role in clogging the arteries that feed the heart. This may explain why more heart attacks are seen in people at high-risk for coronary heart disease (even those with a normal lipid profile) after major holidays, such as the period between Christmas and New Year's. During that period, people tend to overindulge, and holiday foods tend to be heavily laden with bad fats.

So it makes perfect sense to first bring your body back to optimal physiological condition, with a healthy pH of 7.4 in the tissue fluids, to increase the body's alkaline reserve, which can neutralize the acid products after animal protein digestion and stabilize the acid-alkaline balance in the tissue fluids. Second, boost your immune system and restrain the inflammatory response in tissues, including artery walls where fatty plaques are formed. Third, control free radical attacks, which increase after heavy meals, to reduce oxidative reactions in the body, including LDL oxidation. You can then take advantage of your body's natural protection against diseases and self-healing power to either prevent a heart attack or enhance the benefits of treatment (see chapter 6). In fact, I used to belong to this high-risk for coronary heart disease group in the late nineteen nineties; by following this whole-body approach, I have said good-bye to hypertension, and my lipid profile is normal.

This whole-body approach to slowing down the aging process is good for the heart. What is good for the heart tends to be good for the brain, because unobstructed blood vessels will also supply sufficient oxygen and nutrients to your brain. With a healthy cardiovascular system and proper supplementation of essential and special nutrients and proper antioxidants for the brain, you can protect your brain and keep it healthy (see chapter 9).

By bringing your body back to optimal physiological condition, with a healthy pH of 7.4 in tissue fluids, and by changing your lifestyle as well as modifying your nutritional profile with proper supplementation and avoiding certain medications known to cause osteoporosis, you can also improve bone health and prevent osteoporosis (see chapter 7).

This approach may also be good for reducing the risk of age-related cancers. Generally speaking, it takes many years for normal epithelial cells to become precancerous dysplastic cells and to progress to cancer cells after carcinogenic or free radical attacks, depending on which type of cancer. Thus the burden is on us to safeguard our bodies from developing cancer. In fact, 90 percent of human bodies carry precancerous dysplastic cells. If the body's immune system is in optimal condition, immune cells can recognize these cells as foreign invaders and get rid of them before they progress to cancer cells. For those who develop cancer, I would say that their bodies have been allowed to create a "perfect-storm" condition that permits dysplastic cells to progress to cancer cells and then to proliferate. This condition includes (1) increased carcinogenic or free radical attacks, which, in turn, increase the number of precancerous dysplastic cells; (2) a weakened immune system, which allows dysplastic cells to progress to cancer cells; and (3) acidic tissue fluids, in which cancer cells can grow well. Fortunately, we do have some control over these three conditions and thus the ability to reduce the risk of developing age-related cancer. I will discuss this further in chapter 8.

Remember, a "whole-body" approach, in which the whole body works together synergistically to protect your health so you are healthier and live longer, helps you reduce the risks of cardiovascular disease, osteoporosis, age-related cancer, and loss of cognitive ability.

# Chapter 3
# Nutritional Needs for Optimal Immune Function

When healthy, our bodies are capable of inactivating or destroying foreign invaders. Our bodies are also equipped with a healing system designed to handle almost any kind of infection or ill-health. When faced with foreign invaders, the body marshals its army of white blood cells, including natural killer cells, T and B lymphocytes, leucocytes, plasma cells, and macrophages, as well as antibodies and other chemical substances that can kill invaders. These cells work together to ward off infection and to repair damage done by foreign agents. This complicated cellular activity constitutes the body's immune system, with its natural defenses against diseases and self-healing powers.

In order for the immune system to function optimally, our body needs sufficient amounts of essential nutrients, including eight essential and two semi-essential amino acids (from protein-containing foods), two essential fatty acids (omega-3 and omega-6), thirteen kinds of vitamins, and sixteen kinds essential minerals and trace elements, none of which our body can manufacture, meaning they must come from foods or supplements.

We may not *be* what we eat, but our good health irrevocably *depends* on what we eat. The key to good health lies in eating the right amounts of the most beneficial foods for our bodies. Healthful diets include generous amounts of fresh vegetables and fruits, the right amounts of lean proteins, fatty acids (especially marine omega-3 fatty acids), and complex carbohydrates with plenty of fiber, plus quality water.

Following World War II, one of the rewards of prosperity in the United States was a plentiful food supply. With an increase in refined sugar, red meat, and saturated fat, the American diet became richer in calories. Fast foods and processed snack foods loaded with saturated and trans fats became popular; at the same time, technological advances made life more sedentary. As a result, Americans began to put on extra pounds, and they also experienced a rise in cardiovascular disease, diabetes, osteoporosis, and age-related cancer.

## Healthful Diet for Optimal Immune Function

Although nutritional requirements for the immune system vary greatly depending on age, gender, physique, and individual health profiles, all of us need the same basic components of a healthy diet: complete protein, containing all eight essential and two semi-essential amino acids; fat, containing two essential fatty acids; carbohydrates, containing complex carbohydrates and fiber; all thirteen vitamins; and minerals, including sixteen essential minerals and trace elements.

Protein and fat provide building materials for the construction of the whole body, as well as for the production of enzymes, antibodies, and hormones to sustain our life. Fat and carbohydrates provide the calories that supply the body's energy. Vitamins and minerals are essential for the development and growth of our body, as well as the immune system. The key to good health with optimal immune function lies in eating the best, most healthful foods in the right amounts.

**Protein**. The human body begins as a single cell, a fertilized ovum. By adulthood, it consists of 100 trillion cells that are mainly made of protein. So our body must have a continuous supply of protein to sustain life. Protein is essential for the growth and repair of body tissues, including internal organs, muscles, bone, cartilage, skin, and blood, as well as for the formation of hormones, enzymes, and antibodies. Protein is also the primary substance used to replace worn out or dead cells: the lining cells of gastrointestinal tract are replaced every four days; most white blood cells, every ten days; and skin cells, every twenty-four days.

Foods from animal sources, such as meat, chicken, fish, eggs, cheese, and milk provide complete protein that contains all the essential amino acids; protein from vegetables, fruits, nuts, and beans does not contain all the essential amino acids and is therefore known as incomplete protein.

Complete proteins are composed of twenty-two amino acids that are vital for health. Eight amino acids are essential and two are semi-essential; our body either cannot synthesize these or synthesizes them in insufficient amounts. The remaining twelve amino acids can be synthesized by the adult body; after digestion, protein is absorbed by the intestinal tract as amino acid molecules.

When you plan your daily diet, you need to provide a fresh supply of complete protein containing all eight essential and both semi-essential amino acids every day from fish, egg whites, or skinless chicken or turkey breast; because protein, unlike fat and carbohydrate, cannot be stored in your body. Adequate intake for men ranges from sixty-five to eighty grams of protein daily, and women need at least fifty-five grams, depending on height, weight, and level of physical activity.

Unlike fat and carbohydrates, protein cannot be stored in the body for later use. If protein intake exceeds what your body needs, the kidneys process the excess amino acids into ammonia, which is acidic and potentially toxic to the central nervous system. The liver quickly converts ammonia into urea, which is incorporated into urine. During these processes, more acid products are generated. If this occurs frequently and persistently, these endogenous acid products may tilt the pH of tissue fluids toward acidity.

Conversely, insufficient amounts of protein intake over a long period of time will prompt the body to break down its own muscle tissue and transport the amino acids from the destroyed muscle tissue to the more vital organs to sustain life, leading to emaciation. This extreme condition is usually seen in people during famine and also in some terminal cancer patients. Therefore, adequate amounts of complete-protein intake are essential for good health.

Consuming too much protein may have negative repercussions, leading to developing osteoporosis and certain age-related cancers. I will discuss this further in chapters 7 and 8.

**Fat.** Fats are as crucial to a healthy body as protein is; the brain is itself 60 percent fat. Fat is comprised of fatty acids or lipids, which can be saturated, monounsaturated, or polyunsaturated. Trans fats are hydrogenated polyunsaturated fatty acids, manufactured to extend the shelf life of foods; they do not occur naturally. The more hydrogen a fatty acid contains, the more saturated the fat is. Fully hydrogenated trans fats, the "fattest fats," are more saturated than saturated fat. They are very pro-inflammatory—in fact, the most damaging fats of all.

Polyunsaturated fats have multiple reactive sites and are easily oxidized, becoming rancid, then producing lipid peroxides (rancid fats) that are toxic and proinflammatory. Lipid peroxides create massive inflammation in your body when ingested.

Trans fats have a much longer shelf life and do not transfer flavor from one food to another after reuse. This is why trans fats have been used to cook french fries and other fast foods and are still being used in many restaurants today. Commercial baked foods also often contain trans fats as a preservative. They benefit the food manufacturers but are bad for public health. In the United States, California was the first state to partially ban the use of trans fats in restaurants in 2010. Restaurants were allowed to use trans fats in cake batter and to deep fry yeast dough until Jan. 1, 2011.

Dietary fat helps transport the fat-soluble vitamins A, D, E, and K so that they can be absorbed and utilized by the body. The key to good health lies in sufficiently eating the most beneficial fats. Those fats are marine omega-3 fatty acids, which are essential for healthy cellular growth, metabolic function, brain and nerve tissue function, and immune function. They must be provided, because the body cannot manufacture them.

Both omega-3 and omega-6 fatty acids are essential for maintaining fluidity and stability in cell membranes. There are two specific forms of omega-3 fatty acids: DHA and EPA. DHA omega-3 fatty acid is the main structural fatty acid in the gray matter of the brain and retina of the eye. It is essential for brain and eye function. EPA omega-3 fatty acid can reduce blood clotting and restrain the inflammatory response in tissues.

Fatty acids also affect blood cholesterol and triglyceride levels. Saturated fat tends to raise the total blood cholesterol level. Monounsaturated fatty acid (omega-9), found in olive oil, can raise levels of high-density lipoprotein (HDL) cholesterol, without significantly raising overall cholesterol levels. Polyunsaturated fatty acids (omega-3 and omega-6) can lower overall cholesterol levels, but at the expense of HDL levels.

In fact, cholesterol, a fat-like substance, is absolutely essential to our good health and is necessary for our bodies to function normally. It is used in the body as a building block for our hormones and many complex chemicals. Every cell in the body requires cholesterol. The human body makes 80 percent of its cholesterol from fats, protein, and certain carbohydrates, mainly within the liver. The remaining 20 percent comes from dietary sources. The human body synthesizes about 3,000 to 4,000 mg of cholesterol per day and uses cholesterol to manufacture vital hormones, including pituitary hormones, adrenal hormones, DHEA, pregnenolone, aldosterone, testosterone, and estrogen. The brain uses cholesterol to make neurotransmitters that conduct nerve impulses throughout the body. Cholesterol is an important building block for the insulation around nerves, which ensure that nerve impulses are conducted appropriately.

At a time when prime time television commercials for cholesterol-lowering statins promoted by pharmaceutical companies are unrealistically vigorous and high-pressure, it's also important to know the scientific information regarding cholesterol in relation to human health, so that you don't improperly "cholesterol-proof" your body or those of your children. In fact, there is evidence that a low total cholesterol level, below 180 mg/dl, is associated with a high risk of death in older people (*Lancet*, August 2001; *Journal of the American Geriatrics Society*, July 2003) and low LDL cholesterol levels, below 80 mg/dl, with a higher risk of bleeding stroke (*Circulation*, April 2009). This may also help explain why when statin-type drugs oversuppress the production of endogenous cholesterol by the liver cells, memory loss or nerve damage may result (see chapter 6).

Americans consume far too much saturated fat and omega-6 fatty acids and are deficient in marine omega-3 fatty acids. The ratio of omega-6 to omega-3 fatty acids obtained through the average American diet is more like 20:1, while the ideal healthy ratio is around 2:1. This imbalance plus excess intake of saturated fat and trans fat may encourage the development of cardiovascular disease and certain age-related cancers. This will be discussed in chapters 6 and 8.

Fat is higher in calories than any other calorie sources. There are nine calories per gram of fat, as compared to four calories per gram of carbohydrate or protein, meaning that even if you consume a smaller amount of fat, you actually consume more calories. Restricting your intake of fat to the optimum level should help reduce your daily total calories and may help you lose weight.

**Carbohydrates**. There are two kinds of carbohydrates: simple and complex.

Simple carbohydrates are sugars and are found in refined sugars, like candies and snacks, and fruits. Refined sugars are considered the "bad" carbohydrates, because they tend to promote a "sugar rush," a burst of energy that tends to increase the blood glucose level. Ingesting excess refined sugar causes a quick rise in blood glucose, which can attach to the collagen fibers in our skin and other parts of our body through a process known as glycosylation, causing inflammation throughout our bodies. This generalized inflammation, if persistent, produces enzymes that break down collagen, causing the loss of skin elasticity and leading to stiff joints (Perricone, N., *The Perricone Prescription*. Harper-Collins, 2002).

Complex carbohydrates are starches and are found in nuts, legumes, whole grains, and vegetables. They are digested more slowly and do not give a "sugar rush." They provide a steady source of energy. They supply fuel for the body in the form of glycogen, which is used to produce energy for every cell in the body. Carbohydrates also assist in the metabolism of other nutrients.

The American Heart Association recommends that Americans cut back on refined sugars and increase the amount of complex carbohydrates to approximately 55 percent of the total calories consumed in a day.

Fiber is also classified as a carbohydrate. It comes from the cell walls of plants. When combined with carbohydrates, fibers help slow the absorption of glucose into the bloodstream and may relieve digestive disorders. There are two types of fiber: water-soluble and water-insoluble.

Water-soluble fibers include pectins (found in apples, legumes, citrus fruits, and certain vegetables), gums, and mucilages (found in legumes, and oats). Pectins and gums slow sugar absorption, which can be helpful for people with type II diabetes.

Water-insoluble fibers include lignin, cellulose, and hemicelluloses. They are found in wheat bran, whole grains, and certain vegetables. They can absorb water, and they facilitate the elimination of waste products. The National Cancer Institute recommends that an individual consumes 25 to 35 grams of fiber every day.

**Vitamins**. There are thirteen essential vitamins, which cannot be synthesized by the body and must be obtained from foods or supplements. These vitamins can be divided into two groups:

(1) Water-soluble vitamins, including vitamin C and all the B vitamins

(2) Fat-soluble vitamins, including A, D, E, and K

Fat-soluble vitamins can be stored in the body. Vitamins A and D are stored in the liver for up to six months and can be toxic when taken in large amounts. Water-soluble vitamins cannot be stored in the body in large amounts, and any excess is eliminated in the urine once saturation level is reached. So you need to consume them every day.

Vitamins are organic compounds that are essential for normal growth, development, and metabolism, although in very small amounts. They participate in a variety of life-building processes, including the formation and maintenance of blood cells, hormones, and even the creation of our genetic material. Vitamins are used in the production of energy, but they contain no calories. They are used to make enzymes that work as biologic catalysts, triggering cellular metabolic reactions.

In general, if you eat a balanced and healthful daily diet, with four servings of fruits, five servings of vegetables, plenty of grains, the right amounts of lean proteins and fatty acids, you should get all the nutrients you need through your food. However, for a variety of reasons it's not always easy to eat a balanced and healthful diet. To make up for the lack, take a multivitamin pill and other supplements, such as marine omega-3 soft gels, every day. If you do buy supplements, make sure to purchase from a large and reputable manufacturer. Because nutritional supplements are classified as food products, they are not regulated as medicine. It is not uncommon for some bottles to contain ingredients and even contaminants not listed on the label.

All vitamins are necessary for basic life-sustaining metabolic functions. When vitamins are not present in sufficient quantity, metabolism is impaired or ceases. The deficiency of any one vitamin will cause health problems; the signs and symptoms are associated with that particular vitamin deficiency. These are well covered in many nutrition-related articles and books.

**Minerals**. Minerals are inorganic substances. They are important in the production of hormones and enzymes, in the creation of antibodies, and for keeping the blood and tissue fluids from becoming either too acidic or too alkaline. They are found in red blood cells, all cell membranes, hormones, and enzymes, and they are the catalysts of all bodily processes. All of them are necessary for basic metabolic function.

The body needs some minerals in large amounts, called essential major minerals. The most important essential major minerals include calcium, phosphorus, potassium, sodium, chloride, sulfur, and magnesium.

Other essential minerals, called trace elements, are found in the body in only small amounts but are necessary for good health. The most important trace elements include iron, zinc, selenium, manganese, copper, iodine, chromium, molybdenum, and boron.

Minerals are insoluble substances, and some of them are heavy metals, which can be toxic in excess amounts. Do not take mineral supplements beyond the recommended dosage. Extra minerals, such as iron, may build up in the body or purge the body of other minerals, such as zinc.

Essential major mineral and trace element deficiencies occur much more often than vitamin deficiencies. Those at increased risk for mineral deficiencies are people who eat low-calorie diets; the elderly; vegetarians; pregnant women; those who take certain drugs, including diuretics; and those living in areas where the soil has been depleted of certain minerals, such as selenium and boron.

Sodium is the mineral that we don't need to worry about not getting enough of. In fact, most Americans consume far more than they need. The minimum amount of sodium needed for good health is 116 mg per day, and the average American gets more than 4,000 mg per day. Many studies have found that high consumption of sodium is associated with higher blood pressure. The National Institutes of Health and many experts in the field suggest that sodium intake should not exceed 2,400 mg, about a teaspoon of salt, a day. The easiest way to reduce sodium intake is to decrease consumption of processed and prepackaged foods, because a lot of sodium is used to preserve such products.

Minerals can work either together or against each other. A large intake of one mineral can actually produce a deficiency of another. This is especially true of the trace elements zinc and copper. Too much zinc can purge the body of copper. A copper deficiency can cause nerve damage, resulting in symptoms such as anemia, weakness and numbness in legs and arms, loss of balance and difficulty walking, cognitive or memory impairment, and eventually permanent paralysis.

Doctors at the Southwestern Medical Center reported four patients who all used excessive amounts of denture cream such as Poligrip and Fixodent, both of which contain zinc, and had various nerve-related disorders. Thirty million people in the United States wear dentures and use products like Poligrip. There are probably many hundreds more unreported cases. Poligrip contains 38 mg of zinc per ounce. Some people are using a tube of Poligrip a week, giving them forty to forty-five times the recommended dose of zinc. GlaxoSmithKline's action to stop making and marketing Super Poligrip Original comes as hundreds of lawsuits are poised to go to trial, alleging Poligrip caused nerve damage (reported in the *Associated Press*, February 19, 2010).

Minerals like calcium, phosphorus, and magnesium can enhance the absorption and use of other minerals, and, in fact, they work well together. However, the calcium-phosphorus ratio in the blood must stay constant; thus, intake of calcium and phosphorus should be approximately equal. If you have too much phosphorus in your diet, your body will pull calcium from your bones. This is what happens in people consuming excess carbonated soft drinks and highly processed foods. The former contains 136 mg of phosphorus in one 8-oz can, without calcium. If you "super size" your order, you may consume over 1,000 mg of phosphorus without calcium. Highly processed foods are also high in phosphorus and low in calcium. The use of phosphorus as a food additive, a binding agent that stops microbe growth, without balancing calcium also tilts the calcium-phosphorous ratio toward phosphorous. Excess and prolonged consumption of these drinks and foods can lead to net calcium loss in your bones, resulting in osteoporosis.

All human cells contain magnesium, which is necessary for calcium utilization. The more protein you eat, the more magnesium you need to prevent calcium loss in your bones (see chapter 7).

Although water has no nutritional value, the body cannot survive without it. A person can live without food for weeks; without water, death is imminent after only a few days. Water carries nutrients, antibodies, and hormones to and from cells. It is important in the regulation of body temperature, the conduction of nerve impulses, digestion and absorption, and the maintenance of the immune system. Because our body can store only small amounts of water, we need to keep replenishing our body's water supply. It is important to keep our brain adequately hydrated in order to function properly. It takes only a one percent fluid loss for the body to begin to become dehydrated. Everyone should make the effort to drink around eight 8-oz glasses of water a day, depending on weather and levels of physical activity. You should not substitute coffee or teas for water; caffeinated beverages act as diuretics and may, in fact, increase your need for water.

The water you drink also contributes to the acid-alkaline balance in your tissue fluids. When you drink water from the same source over a long period of time (say, for years), make sure that the water has a pH close to 7.4 and contains the essential minerals your body needs. Water filtered by a reverse osmosis system is acidic and not suitable for long-term drinking because all minerals are removed during membrane filtration. This is true for distilled water, which contains no minerals and is acidic after exposure to air. Water treated by a water softener system contains too much sodium and is also not suitable for drinking. Drinking plenty of good quality water is one of the best and easiest ways to help maintain a healthy body.

As mentioned above, the key to good health lies in eating the right amounts of the most beneficial foods. The general principles for choosing healthful foods follow:

1.  Make vegetables and fruits the major part of your diet.

2.  Eat lean meats and skinless poultry.

3.  Eat nuts, preferably walnuts and almonds.

4.  Eat fatty fish and shell fish.

5.  Eat whole grains.

6. Restrict trans fat, saturated fat, and omega-6 fatty acids (especially corn, sunflower seed and safflower oils).

7. Restrict processed foods.

8. Restrict sodium and sugar.

9. Take vitamin and mineral supplements.

10. Take fish oil soft gels if you don't eat fish several times a week.

11. Take proper antioxidant supplements.

# Chapter 4
# Avoiding Mistakes in Taking Medication

Following reports of the drug-related deaths of Heath Ledger, Michael Jackson, and Brittany Murphy over the past two years, many consumers began to realize that supposedly "safe drugs" could also go terribly wrong.

In fact, unintentional overdoses occur far more often than most consumers imagine. Side effects from non-steroidal anti-inflammatory drugs (NSAIDs) including ibuprofen and aspirin, result in more than 100,000 hospitalizations and thousands of deaths each year in the United States. Prescription drugs for allergies, arthritis, diabetes, and other ailments kill some 200,000 Americans every year (*Vanity Fair*, "Deadly Medicine." January 2011). These deaths and related health problems caused by unintentional overdoses occur in just a tiny fraction of the overall drugs' users (*Journal of American Medical Association*, 226:2847–51, 1991).

This kind of accident may happen to anyone who is uninformed and unaware of potential problems in taking medication, especially when he or she is sick and anxious to get well. Overdoses are common in the following situations:

1. In some drugs, the margin between a safe dose and a potentially lethal one is small. For instance, the maximum safe daily dose of acetaminophen is 4,000 mg. However, a daily dose of 7,000 mg can cause severe liver damage. About 10 percent of acetaminophen-related deaths have occurred at levels between 2,000 and 4,000 mg. People who have liver disease are particularly vulnerable.

2. Sick people who are anxious to get well may take more than the recommended daily dose without realizing it. It is not uncommon that some people don't bother to read the instructions and pop more than the recommended amount. Over-the-counter products are believed to be safe. Prime time television commercials vigorously promoted by pharmaceutical companies play to this false sense of security.

3. It is often difficult for patients to realize that the various medications they are taking for different ailments may contain the same potentially toxic ingredient. Take acetaminophen as an example. It's safe if taken as instructed, but if you take Tylenol for a headache, plus cough syrup three times a day, plus an over-the-counter sleep aid for insomnia, plus Percocet for lower back pain, then you have exceeded the recommended safe dosage, because all these medications have acetaminophen as their main ingredient. Acetaminophen is contained in more than two hundred over-the-counter and prescription products. Even conscientious patients may not be aware of how much acetaminophen is in their prescription pain reliever, because it is often labeled as APAP, an acronym for its chemical name: N-acetyl-para-aminophenol.

4. The liver is the most common site affected by potentially toxic drugs, such as acetaminophen and Neurontin. The first symptoms of acute liver failure caused by an overdose seems like the flu and doesn't set in for several days. Once symptoms set in, it may already be too

late to save one's liver and consequently one's life. Although the liver is capable of regenerating from some injuries, that's not the case with acetaminophen and Neurontin poisoning, in which every cell is being damaged at once.

5. If patients take several kinds of drugs at the same time, they may experience unexpected, adverse cross chemical reactions of these drugs. Some drug effects are enhanced by other drugs, which can lead to serious side effects or even sudden cardiac arrest, liver failure, and/ or kidney failure. For instance, patients taking both a blood thinner, such as coumadin, and acetaminophen preparations have a much higher chance of bleeding. Pepto-Bismol, which contains 2,080 mg of salicylate, may interact with coumadin and increase the risk for bleeding. Arthritis rubs, such as Bengay, Icy Hot Cream, Mentholatum, Deep Heating, and Thera-Gesic, may contain methyl salicylate, and also pose a risk for this interaction. Therefore, care needs to be taken to avoid an accidental overdose and drug-drug interactions.

When incidents of severe side effects caused by certain drugs are due to the consumer's ignorance or misinformation about the dosage in relation to the drugs' side effects, such incidents can be avoided through education. Unfortunately, overdosing on some drugs can cause irreversible tissue damages and may lead to chronic conditions, like drug-induced hepatitis, which will affect the dosage limit of various drugs in the future and also increase vulnerability to adverse drug effects. The accumulation of toxic chemicals increases the toxic burden in the body. The immune system is then compromised or may even be destroyed. It is, therefore, important not to make mistakes while taking medication.

Below are discussions of the side effects of some popular commonplace drugs, based on cases reported in the medical journals. Under the current "high-pressure" marketing and vigorous promotion by pharmaceutical companies on prime time television, consumers need to have some basic knowledge about the proper use and side effects of these widely used drugs in order to avoid mistakes in taking medication that can bring further health problems.

## Acid-Suppressing Drugs

Over-the-counter antacids include Mylanta, Maalox, Tums, Rolaids, and Gaviscon. These drugs can neutralize acid. Another type of over-the-counter acid-blocking medications includes Pepcid-AC, Tagamet, and Zantac. They work by blocking histamine receptors that stimulate gastric acid secretion. These medications do not heal the inflammation of the stomach or esophagus. Among them, magnesium-containing antacids can cause diarrhea, while aluminum-containing ones cause constipation. Prescription medications include proton pump inhibitors such as Prevacid and Prilosec. These medications work by blocking the pump mechanism in the acid-making parietal cells. They are used for severe heartburn and/or gastro-esophageal reflux disease (GERD).

Prolonged use of acid-suppressing drugs can interfere with the absorption of vitamin B-12, calcium, and iron, leading to an increased risk of fractures due to calcium deficiency (*Osteoporosis International*, December 2009), as well as intestinal infection (*American Journal of Gastroenterology*, September 2007) and pneumonia (*Annals of Internal Medicine*, September 2008). Patients with B-12 deficiency from long-term use of antacid drugs may experience irreversible neurological damage. Symptoms include fatigue, confusion, poor memory, depression, and peripheral neuropathy (burning, tingling, and/or numbness in feet and hands).

A rare but disabling side effect is known as tardive dyskinesia; characterized by involuntary, repetitive movements of the extremities, lip smacking, tongue enlargement and protrusion, rapid eye movements, and impaired movement of the fingers. Unfortunately, there is no known treatment for tardive dyskinesia.

If patients abruptly stop taking acid-suppressing drugs, the parietal cells in the gastric mucosa may reactively secrete even more acids, causing severe discomfort. Gradual tapering of the dose over a few weeks may help minimize the unpleasant rebound symptoms.

**Non-Narcotic Analgesics**

This type of drug includes Advil, Motrin, Aleve, Anaprox, Naprosyn, Celebrex, Indocin, Cataflam, Voltaren, Mobic, Nuprin, aspirin, Tylenol, and Nabumetone. Prolonged use or overdose of these medications can result in serious side effects, including stomach upset and bleeding ulcers, hypertension, drowsiness, mental fogginess, blood clots, elevated liver enzymes (due to drug-induced hepatitis, which may lead to liver failure), and kidney failure. Ibuprofen products, such as Advil, Motrin, and Nuprin can affect the mucosa of the stomach, predisposing elderly patients to ulcer disease and major bleeding problems.

Non-steroidal anti-inflammatory drugs (NSAIDs) can cause ringing in the ears (tinnitus) and even hearing loss resulting from damage of the tiny hair cells inside the ear (*Drug Safety*, March 1996). There is no magic bullet to cure ringing in the ears. A recent study suggests that long-term use of acetaminophen is linked with hearing loss, especially in men under fifty years of age (*American Journal of Medicine*, March 2010). According to a study published in the *American Journal of Medicine*, regular use of pain relief medicine appears to increase men's risk of hearing loss: a 33 percent increase for aspirin, 61 percent for ibuprofen, and 99 percent for acetaminophen.

An analysis of nearly twenty studies involving more than 400,000 patients concluded that regular use of acetaminophen is linked to a higher risk of asthma (*Chest*, November 2009). Acetaminophen is contained in more than two hundred over-the-counter and prescription medications, from headache and cold remedies to cough syrup and sleep aids. It's easy to take more than the recommended daily dose without realizing it. Americans purchased more than twenty-eight billion doses of acetaminophen in 2005, and acetaminophen-related liver damage caused 450 deaths and 56,000 emergency room visits a year. Consumers must stay alert to prevent an overdose of acetaminophen.

**Statin-Type Cholesterol-Lowering Drugs**

This type of drug includes Lipitor, Crestor, Zocor, Pravachol, and Mevacor. There are three main side effects of statin-type drugs:

1. Muscle pain, weakness, and cramps

2. Drug-induced hepatitis

3. Memory loss

Some patients may show signs of nerve damage, breathing difficulty, and sexual dysfunction. Memory loss may present as transient global amnesia. Patients cannot continue to work because they cannot do the simple jobs they used to do, such as transferring dollar amounts from hard copy to electronic spreadsheets; they may forget names or ask the same questions all the time. There are more than a hundred reports of Lou Gehrig's disease, which causes muscle paralysis, in people taking statin-type medications.

Statin-type drugs may raise blood sugar levels. A large study of more than 17,000 patients (the Jupiter Trial) reported a higher incidence of diabetes in the subjects taking Crestor (*New England Journal of Medicine*, November 2008).

A large clinical study showed that 3 percent of patients taking a sugar pill or placebo had a heart attack compared to 2 percent of the patients taking Lipitor. Except among high-risk heart patients, the benefits of statins are overstated. An estimated 10 percent to 15 percent of statin users suffer side effects (Carey J., "Do Cholesterol Drugs Do Any Good?" *Business Week*, January 28, 2008).

## Antidepressants

This type of drug includes Prozac, Effexor, Cymbalta, Lexapro, Paxil, and Zoloft. They are prescribed for anxiety, depression, bulimia, chronic fatigue syndrome, obsessive-compulsive disorders, post-menopausal syndrome, and post-traumatic stress disorder. Antidepressants can interfere with sexual functions; they reduce libido, interfere with arousal, block orgasm, and cause erectile dysfunction. A recent study suggests that the sexual side effects may persist indefinitely even after the drugs are discontinued, and there are no antidotes for these side effects (*The Open Psychology Journal*, Vol. 1, 2008).

When patients suddenly stop taking such drugs, they may experience dizziness, headaches, insomnia, anxiety, sweating, visual disturbance, nervousness, and an electrical shock-like sensation ("brain zap"). Gradual tapering of the dose over several months may be the best way to minimize the unpleasant symptoms of withdrawal.

According to a newly released analysis including 718 patients, antidepressants provide relief only in extreme cases but are no more effective than placebo for patients with mild to moderate depression, as rated on the Hamilton Depression Rating Scale (*Journal of the American Medical Association*, January 2010). For some patients, the drugs' side effects may cancel any benefit.

## Bone Density-Enhancing Drugs

This type of drug includes Actonel, Boniva, Fosamax, Reclast, and Evista. These drugs increase bone density by reducing bone breakdown, limiting the release of calcium from bone into the blood.

A surprising number of medicines have a negative effect on bone density, including prednisone, inhaled corticosteroids, like Advair or Flovent, and certain seizure medicines, such as Dilantin, Klonopin, and Tegretol, as well as high-dose thyroid hormones, like Levoxyl or Synthroid. A recent study (*Obstetrics and Gynecology*, January 2010) found that 45 percent of users of the birth control Depo-Provera experienced bone mineral density loss of 5 percent or more in the hip or lower spine within two years.

There is a growing controversy over osteoporosis drugs. There are many reports of low-trauma fractures of the thigh bone or other major bones occurring in users. Furthermore, due to the slowing bone turnover, there can be delayed healing or complete failure of a fracture to heal. Although all these drugs have been shown to reduce the risk of osteoporotic fractures during clinical trials, none comes even close to preventing them. These drugs intended to strengthen bones might actually cause fractures instead (*New England Journal of Medicine*, March 2008). At the 2010 annual meeting of the American Academy of Orthopedic Surgeons, researchers presented data suggesting that after four or five years of treatment by these drugs, some bone may lose its structural integrity and become brittle.

Long-term use of Actonel, Boniva, Fosamax, and Reclast may suppress bone turnover and lead to serious complications, such as severe and incapacitating bone, joint, and muscle pain, as well as thigh bone fracture (*JAMA*, February 2009). There are case reports of jawbone necrosis (osteonecrosis of the jaw) triggered by such osteoporosis drugs (*Journal of the American Dental Association*, January 2009). About 4 percent of Fosamax users experienced this serious complication (*New England Journal of Medicine*, March, 2008). Other side effects include difficulty swallowing, esophagitis, gastric ulcer, atrial fibrillation, and a possible increased risk of esophageal cancer (*New England Journal of Medicine*, January 2009).

A recent study showed that increasing the alkaline content of the diet by eating more fruits and vegetables to increase the body's alkaline reserve can be used as a safe and low-cost approach to preventing osteoporosis and improving bone health, without adverse effects (*Journal of Clinical Endocrinology and Metabolism*, January 2009).

## Blood Pressure-Lowering Drugs

Commonly used anti-hypertensive medications fall into five categories:

1. **Diuretics** like hydrochrothiazide, including Lasix, Aldactone, Esidrex, and Dyrenium. These medications cause the body to eliminate sodium, accompanied by water loss; thus, excess fluid is excreted. During the process of treatment, two other important minerals, potassium and magnesium, may also be depleted. Prolonged use may cause adverse side effects, such as gout, elevated blood fats, impotence, and gynecomastia. Loss of potassium and magnesium can cause dizziness, fatigue, and muscle cramping. Side effects can be managed by adjusting the dosage.

2. **Beta blockers** include such drugs as Inderal, Tenormin, Lopressor, Normodyne, Corgard, Visken, and Blocadren. All these medications act to block the action of adrenalin at the beta receptors, in order to slow down the heart rate. The medications of this class may cause some side effects, including fatigue, dizziness, swelling of feet and ankles, and shortness of breath from constricting the airways in the lungs. When patients stop taking the medication abruptly, they may experience a dramatic rise in blood pressure, occasionally to dangerously high levels. Stopping a beta blocker safely requires the careful tapering of the dose.

3. **Alpha blockers** include such drugs as Cardura, Minipress, and Hytrin. These medications relax the muscular layer of the arteries, allowing them to dilate, thereby dropping the blood pressure, but their effectiveness may wane with time. They tend to cause unpleasant side effects, including severe hypotension, heart palpitation, headache, fainting, and nervous agitation.

4. **Angiotensin-converting enzyme (ACE) inhibitors** include such drugs as Lotensin, Capoten, Vasolec, Monopril, Lisinopril, Accupril, Altace, and Mavik. The ACE inhibitors prevent blood vessel constriction

by stopping the conversion of the angiotensin I into the powerful blood vessel constrictor angiotensin II. The side effects include dry cough, dizziness, hypotension, alterations in taste, swelling, erectile dysfunction, and generalized muscle weakness. The persistent dry cough is sometimes so severe that the patient cannot lie down to sleep without gagging. Up to one-third of patients taking ACE inhibitors may experience chronic cough (*Chest Supplement*, January 2006).

5. **Calcium channel blockers** include such drugs as Carizen, Norvasc, Procardia, Plendil, Cardene, and Adalat. This class of medications prevents blood vessel constriction by blocking excessive calcium flooding through the calcium channel. Side effects include headache, slow heart rate, fluid swelling, dizziness, gastrointestinal distress, and occasionally heart palpitations.

**Blood Glucose-Lowering Drugs**

Oral medications that lower blood glucose for patients with type II diabetes fall into four categories:

1. Sulfonylureas include such drugs as Orinase, Diabinese, Tolinase, Dymalor, DiaBeta, Glucotrol, and Amaryl. These drugs work by stimulating the pancreas to release more stored insulin. A common side effect is hypoglycemia.

2. Metformin. This drug improves insulin sensitivity, reducing the release of glucose from the liver and increasing its uptake by muscles. Patients with liver or kidney disease cannot take this drug because of the risk of lactic acidosis (excessive amounts of lactic acid in the blood), a potentially fatal complication. This drug may induce weight loss; therefore, it is especially useful for obese diabetics. It may be associated with an increased risk of vitamin B-12 deficiency (*Archives of Internal Medicine*, October 2006). Two other drugs, Avandia and Actos, that also improve insulin sensitivity may induce weight gain and increase LDL and risk of heart attack. According to a recent investigation by the government (reported in the *New York Times*, February 21, 2010),

Avandia was linked to 304 heart-related deaths during the third quarter of 2009.

3. Acarbose. This drug inhibits the action of digestive enzymes, alpha glucosidases, so as to slow the breakdown of sucrose and starches. Side effects include severe flatulence, diarrhea, and abdominal cramping.

4. Troglitazone. This drug also increases insulin sensitivity. Concern has been raised about the possibility of harmful liver effects. Therefore, liver enzymes should be measured every month for the first six months of treatment.

## Sleep Aids and Medications

In general, sleep medications are most effective when used sparingly for short-term situations, such as travel across many time zones or recovering from a medical procedure. Unfortunately, sleep medications don't cure insomnia, and they can often make the problem worse in the long run. For people with chronic insomnia, a good sleep environment, behavioral techniques, stress relief, and relaxation provide relief without the risk of medication side effects or tolerance problems. Concerns about the use of both over-the-counter and prescription sleep medications should be seriously considered.

1. Side effects. Over-the-counter sleep aids, such as Advil PM, Nytol, Somiflex, Benadryl, and Tylenol PM, contain the sedating antihistamine diphenhydramine. The common side effects include next-day drowsiness, unsteadiness, confusion, forgetfulness, dry mouth, dizziness, and urinary retention.

2. Drug tolerance. Over time, in order to get the sleep medication to work, you may have to take more and more drugs, which can lead to an unending cycle that includes additional side effects.

3. Drug dependence. Once you start to rely on the medication for sleep, you may be unable to sleep without it.

4. Withdrawal symptoms. If you stop the medication abruptly, you may experience withdrawal symptoms, such as sweating, nausea, and shaking.

5. Drug interactions. Sleep medications can interact with other drugs, which can be dangerous in combination with some prescription pain killers and sedatives.

When we introduce a foreign substance, such as a pharmacologic agent, to our body, its benefit often ends when we stop using the product; however, it may induce a host of negative side effects that can persist for a variable length of time.

First, some of the drugs we take work by "blocking" or "inhibiting" certain physiological processes or functions in the body. They are intended to circumvent certain physiological processes or functions in only one particular site; however, many other unintended sites may also be involved, leading to the unfortunate phenomenon of curing one problem and developing another.

Second, certain ingredients, such as acetaminophen, contained in many drugs are potentially toxic, and the immune system will react to these substances once they are absorbed by the body. The liver is the detoxification center in our body. The lining cells of liver sinusoids, known as Kupffer cells, are the first line of defense in fighting off toxic substances. However, prolonged use or overdosage of these medicines can deplete the protective Kupffer cells, resulting in injury to liver cells, drug-induced hepatitis, or liver failure. The accumulation of toxic chemicals from pharmaceuticals increases the toxic burden in our body. The immune system is then compromised or may even be destroyed.

Third, a surprising number of medicines have a negative effect on vitamin and mineral absorption, leading to deficiencies. For instance, prolonged use of acid-suppressing drugs can interfere with vitamin B-12, calcium, and iron absorption. Medication containing excess zinc (such as zinc cough drops and Poligrip) can purge the body of copper, which is an essential trace element. Certain medications, such as steroids and anticonvulsants, are known to have a serious negative effect on bone mineral density, and evidence is emerging with regard to other drugs (see chapter 7).

Fourth, some drugs are composed of acids that strongly acidify after being absorbed by the body; prolonged use of these drugs may upset the acid-alkaline balance in the tissue fluids, and, in turn, affect the efficiency of some physiological functions taking place in intracellular and extracellular tissue fluids, leading to more health problems.

These are the reasons why drugs' adverse effects can build up over time to become life-threatening health problems. There are many such case reports published in the *Peoples' Pharmacy* and health journals. Often patients started taking one medication for a minor health problem; along the way, they developed side effects for which they were given more medications. Over time, more complicated, serious health problems emerged, requiring even more medications. In the process, the body's natural protection against diseases and self-healing powers were being derailed by medications, not helped.

If we instead take the course of strengthening our body with health-promoting, nutritional substances that are natural to the body, we reap genuine health benefits with few adverse effects, if any. The caveat is that the results may be gradual, not immediate.

In dire situations medications can be lifesaving, and there are many happy reports of cancer remissions and successful management of ailments. In the age of "the informed patient," it is up to us, with the help of health professionals, to be our own advocates and not to be influenced by "high-pressure" marketing and vigorous promotions by pharmaceutical companies. Avoiding mistakes in taking medication is also essential to maintaining your good health.

Drugs can work both for and against us. Understand their properties and make sure that you know how to use them properly.

1. Always read the instructions, especially the contraindications, carefully before you take the medication.

2. If you take several medications, care needs to be taken to avoid an accidental overdose and drug-to-drug interaction.

3. If the drug you take is for long-term use, discuss the possible adverse side effects with your doctor.

# Chapter 5
## Wise Use of Antioxidants

An antioxidant is a chemical substance that protects body cells against the adverse effects of free radicals, which damage cells and tissue and play a role in heart disease, age-related cancer, and neurodegenerative diseases. A free radical is as deadly as a germ, but in a different way. Neither one germ nor one free radical presents a grave danger by itself. When free radicals create chain reactions, they cause damage over time.

Antioxidants work by preventing the oxidative damage induced by free radicals. They can donate an electron to a free radical without harm to themselves, thus putting an end to the destructive damage of cells and tissues. In our body, the work of an antioxidant is comparable to stopping a sliced apple from browning, which is also an oxidative reaction. If you dip the cut apple in orange or lemon juice, which contain vitamin C, an antioxidant, it stays white.

Oxidative reactions can produce free radicals that start chain reactions, damaging considerably more cells. Antioxidants terminate these chain reactions by removing free radicals and inhibit other oxidative reactions by being oxidized themselves. Antioxidants can be reducing agents, such as ascorbic acid or polyphenols. They are found in many foods, including fruits, vegetables, nuts, grains, and some meats, poultry, and fish. Processed foods contain fewer antioxidants than fresh and uncooked foods, since the preparation processes may expose the food to oxygen.

Antioxidants are widely used in the food industry as food additives to help guard against food deterioration. The most common foods attacked by oxidation are unsaturated fats, and oxidation causes them to turn rancid. They are usually preserved by salting, smoking, or fermenting. Less fatty foods, like fruits, are sprayed with sulfurous antioxidants prior to air drying. Oxidation is often catalyzed by metals. This is why fats, such as butter, should never be kept in metal containers or wrapped in aluminum foil. Some fatty foods, including olive oil, are partially protected by their natural antioxidants, which increase their shelf life. Antioxidant preservatives are also added to lipid-based cosmetics, such as moisturizers and lipstick, to prevent rancidity.

Although oxidative reactions are inevitable over the course of a life, they can be damaging because of the free radicals produced. If our body is low in antioxidants and cannot counteract the free radical attacks, oxidative stress will result. The brain, which is 60 percent fats, is uniquely vulnerable to oxidative injuries, due to its high metabolic rate and elevated levels of polyunsaturated fats (including omega-3 and omega-6 fatty acids), the target of lipid peroxidation. Oxidative stress is thought to contribute to the development of a wide range of neurodegenerative diseases, including Parkinson's disease and Alzheimer's disease. Antioxidants are now being investigated as preventive measures against oxidative stress in neurons and as possible treatments for neurodegenerative diseases.

In animal experiments, a low calorie intake extends lifespan, which is thought to be due to a reduction in oxidative stress. Nevertheless, antioxidant supplements do not appear to increase life expectancy in humans.

Antioxidants are now widely available as dietary supplements used in the hope of maintaining health and preventing diseases, including coronary heart disease and age-related cancer. Initial studies suggested that some antioxidant supplements might promote health. In a large study in France, over 12,500 men and women took either low-dose antioxidants, including ascorbic acid, vitamin E, beta carotene, selenium, and zinc, or placebo pills for an average of 7.5 years (*Archives of Internal Medicine*, 164:2335-42, 2004). The investigators found there was no statistically significant effect of the antioxidants on overall survival, cancer, or heart disease. Such contradictory findings and reports seem to point to some other contributing factors involved in the pathogenesis of such chronic diseases, and using antioxidants alone, especially at the low dosage used in the French study, cannot prevent those diseases. It becomes clear that any one measure or a few supplements do not guarantee any protective effect against coronary heart disease and age-related cancer.

**Adverse Effects of Antioxidants**

Very high doses of some antioxidants may have harmful effects. The Beta-Carotene and Retinol Trial study of lung cancer patients found that smokers given high doses of beta-carotene and vitamin A had increased rates of lung cancer (*Journal of National Cancer Institute*, 88:1550–1559, 1996). Subsequent studies confirmed the results of this trial (*American Journal of Clinical Nutrition*, June 1999).

While antioxidant supplements are widely used in attempts to prevent the development of cancer, research has found that antioxidants may interfere with cancer treatments. Since the environment of cancer cells causes high levels of oxidative stress, these cancer cells are more susceptible to further oxidative stress induced by chemotherapy and/ or radiotherapy, leading to cancer cell death. Antioxidant supplements can decrease the effectiveness of treatments by reducing the oxidative stress in cancer cells (*Cancer Research*, August 2003). On the other hand, other reviews have shown that antioxidants could reduce side effects of chemotherapy and/or radiotherapy, simply because very high levels of free radicals are created throughout the body during treatment (*International Journal of Cancer*, September 2008).

## Wise Use of Antioxidants

As mentioned above, oxidative reactions are inevitable during the course of life, but they leave a trail of free radicals, which start chain reactions that can damage cells and tissues, giving rise to many diseases. In a healthy body, an adequate level of antioxidants can terminate these chain reactions and eliminate the presence of oxidative stress. Therefore, we, especially seniors, need to increase the level of antioxidants in our body by taking supplements because the endogenous antioxidants decrease as we age. In view of the harmful effects caused by some antioxidants, wise use of antioxidants is essential.

Our body makes endogenous antioxidant enzymes, such as superoxide dismutase, coenzyme Q10 (CoQ10), and alpha lipoic acid, but quantities decrease substantially with age, and we have to replenish them from foods and nutritional supplements.

There are several thousand research articles in the literature about the values of antioxidants. Wise use of antioxidants may help our body control free radical attacks without causing harmful effects. As noted in chapter 2, there are four main categories of supplemental antioxidants: vitamins, minerals, chemicals, and hormones. The remainder of this chapter will provide a more in-depth look at some of the key antioxidants in each category:

## Antioxidant Vitamins

**Vitamin A:** There are two varieties of antioxidants in the vitamin A family, which also includes its precursors, carotenoids. Vitamin A, known as retinol or retinyl, is always found in animal products, such as liver, milk, eggs, cream, butter, and fish liver oil. Vitamin A helps maintain protective barriers against infectious organisms entering the body by preserving the integrity of the skin and mucous membranes, and it is vital to the health of our immune system.

As reported by the United Nations Children's Fund (UNICEF), vitamin A deficiency affects about one hundred million children worldwide. A dozen field studies indicate that supplementing the diets of children at risk of vitamin A deficiency saved lives that would otherwise be taken by diarrhea, malaria, and measles. Supplementation also reduced the incidence of pregnancy-related deaths among women by 44 percent and deaths from diarrhea by 35 to 50 percent. The number of deaths due to measles was reduced by half, a consequence thought to stem from vitamin A's crucial effect on the function of the immune system.

A contrary view in the *New England Journal of Medicine* holds that women who take large doses of vitamin A around the time of conception or early in their pregnancy run a higher risk of delivering infants with birth defects (*New England Journal of Medicine*, November 1995). No matter what, vitamin A is essential for normal cellular differentiation and in regulating organ development in the fetus. The researchers recommended that pregnant women either limit their vitamin A consumption to 2,500 IU daily or, alternatively, take beta-carotene instead, which is only converted into vitamin A when the body needs it, therefore eliminating potential toxicity problems.

When vitamin A levels in the body are moderate, it works as an antioxidant. However, when you overdose the supplement, the surplus vitamin does the opposite. High doses of vitamin A oxidize tissues, cause DNA damage, and deplete your bones of calcium. Although it is important to get sufficient vitamin A, too much vitamin A can actually be harmful (Roizen, M. F., *The Real Age Makeover*. Collin, 2004).

**Carotenoids:** Over 600 different carotenoids have been identified. Only forty to fifty, however, are found in the American diet, and only about fourteen are actually found in the bloodstream. The major carotenoids include beta-carotene, lycopene, alpha-carotene, cryptoxanthin, bioflavonoids, and lutein. Virtually all carotenoids work as antioxidants to rid the body of cell-damaging free radicals. High blood levels of carotenoids are found to be associated with a lower risk of chronic degenerative diseases and appear to enhance the immune system and protect against age-related ailments, such as stroke and heart disease.

**Beta-carotene:** Beta-carotene, the most commonly seen carotenoid, is converted to vitamin A inside the body; however, the amount of vitamin A converted depends on the body's need. Beta-carotenes are found in carrots, tomatoes, sweet potatoes, and dark green vegetables, such as broccoli, kale, and spinach, and yellow and orange fruits such as papaya, apricots, and melons. People with hypothyroidism or diabetes may not be able to efficiently convert beta-carotene to vitamin A and may assume a yellowish pigmentation in the skin around the abdomen area. The pigmentation is not harmful and will fade once beta-carotene intake is stopped. Beta-carotene limits oxidative reactions by neutralizing free radicals inside the cells and protects lipoproteins against oxidative damage, thus reducing the risk of cardiovascular disease.

**Lycopene:** Lycopene, found in tomatoes, guava, watermelon, apricots, and pink grapefruit, reduces the risk of certain cancers and cardiovascular diseases. Harvard University researchers found that the men who had the greatest amounts of lycopene in their diet (6.5 mg per day) showed a 21 percent decreased risk of prostate cancer. In fact, lycopene is the most abundant carotenoid in the prostate, and high blood levels of lycopene have been linked to prostate cancer prevention. Conversely, prostate cancer patients have been reported to have low levels of lycopene in both blood and prostate tissue. In Europe, researchers have also found a statistically significant association between high dietary lycopene and a 48 percent lower risk of cardiovascular disease (*American*

*Journal of Epidemiology*, 146:618–626, 1997). A clinical trial showed that lycopene supplementation had boosted immune function and 15 mg of lycopene per day increased natural killer cell activity by 28 percent in twelve weeks.

Among other members of the carotenoid family, **alpha-carotene** is found in pumpkin, cantaloupe, carrots, yellow and red peppers, and corn. It may inhibit the proliferation of skin, liver, and lung cancer cells. **Cryptoxanthin** is found in peaches, tangerines, oranges, papaya, and nectarines. Studies showed that high blood levels of cryptoxanthin were associated with a significant reduction in cervical cancer risk. **Bioflavonoids** are found in onions, buckwheat, most fruits, including plums, grapes, apples, cherries, and in the white rind of citrus fruits. They decrease the risk of cardiovascular disease and some cancers and enhance the effects of vitamin C. **Lutein** is found in spinach, mustard, broccoli, kale, and hot chilies. It is known for preventing age-related macular degeneration, an eye disease that can result in blindness.

**Vitamin C:** Vitamin C is one of the most widely heralded antioxidants. One of its most important functions is the synthesis, formation, and maintenance of a protein-like substance called collagen that supports and holds tissues and organs together to sustain life. Vitamin C is a potent broad-spectrum virus fighter when used in large doses. Vitamin C helps keep the arteries clear by inhibiting oxidation of fat in the walls of blood vessels. It converts cholesterol to a form that can be washed out of the body easily, thereby inhibiting lipid buildup.

Many large-scale population studies showed statistically significant reduction in the risk of virtually all kinds of cancer with a high intake of vitamin C. Most animals produce between 10,000 and 20,000 mg of vitamin C every day in their bodies. They do have a stronger immune system, and they do not have heart attacks. Humans do not produce vitamin C in their bodies and must obtain it from outside sources. However, vitamin C is easily destroyed by light and air, and is absent in most cooked, canned foods and fruits. You may lack sufficient vitamin

C to ward off colds, prevent cancer and other diseases, even when you think you have taken sufficient vitamin C.

**Vitamin E:** Vitamin E (d-alpha tocopherol) is a powerful antioxidant that seems to have a number of immune-protective and immune-stimulating effects. Hundreds of studies have shown that the higher the intake of vitamin E, the less likely the risk of cancer. One study in the *British Journal of Cancer* reported that the group of 5,000 women with the lowest blood serum levels of vitamin E had four to five times the risk of developing breast cancer, stomach cancer, cancer of the pancreas, and cancer of the urinary tract. Most authorities agree that a person should take 400 to 800 IUs of vitamin E from natural d-alpha tocopherol (not synthetic dl-alpha tocopherol) daily. However, if you have high blood pressure, your intake should not be more than 800 IUs, due to its blood thinning property. Do not take vitamin E in combination with aspirin, which may increase the risk of bleeding.

**Antioxidant Minerals**

**Zinc:** Zinc is an important antioxidant mineral that specifically promotes T-lymphocyte immunity. It is found in oysters, herring, wheat germ, pumpkin seeds, milk, crab, lobster, pork, beef, chicken, turkey, liver, and eggs. It promotes wound healing and helps slow down the progression of macular degeneration. People with low zinc levels have been found to have lowered resistance to disease, an atrophied thymus gland with a reduced number of T-lymphocytes, and impotence. Fingernails with white spots or bands or an opaquely white appearance are a sign of zinc deficiency. More than two hundred enzymes in our body, including the enzymes involved in the production of nucleic acids DNA and RNA, require zinc for their activity. Zinc also plays a role in the structure and function of cell membranes.

The recommended dosage is 10 to 15 mg daily, accompanied by copper at a zinc: copper ratio of 10:1. Daily intake should not exceed 30 mg. Too much zinc can damage the immune system. If you take six zinc-containing cough lozenges (the recommended maximum dosage per day) for a total of 80 mg, you'll have too much zinc in your body, which can trigger the loss of copper. Following a 2008 report in the medical journal *Neurology* about a possible link between zinc found in denture-cream and nerve damage, doctors at the Southwestern Medical Center reported four patients suffering various nerve-related disorders, all of whom had used excessive amounts of Poligrip and Fixodent, which have zinc in their formula. The human body needs zinc and copper in the proper amounts. Too much zinc can purge the body of copper. A copper deficiency causes nerve damage, resulting in symptoms such as anemia, weakness, and numbness in legs and arms, loss of balance and difficulty walking, cognitive or memory impairment, and eventually permanent paralysis.

**Selenium**: Selenium is a powerful antioxidant that stimulates antibody response to germ infections and enhances the effects of vitamin E. It is found in organ meats, seafood, brewer's yeast, onions, garlic, mushrooms, wheat germ, and some whole grains. Selenium and vitamin E work together synergistically, and they work best when taken together. In some studies, antibody response increased as much as thirtyfold when these two supplements were taken together. More than 400 articles have documented the role of selenium in cancer prevention. A study by Larry Clark of the University of Arizona, reported in the *Journal of the American Medical Association* showed that taking 200 mcg of selenium for about seven years reduced the occurrence of all cancers in a group of 1,300 older people by 42 percent and cancer deaths by nearly 50 percent, compared with those on a placebo (*JAMA*, December 1996). The recommended dosage is 200 mcg daily as a supplement. Selenium is one of the trace minerals that are not easily excreted by the body, so you should not take more than what is recommended, as high doses may be toxic.

**Manganese**: Manganese is found in whole grains, peas, nuts, green leafy vegetables, beets, egg yolks, bananas, organ meats, and milk. It is required for many enzymatic reactions, bone development, collagen production, and thymus gland function. Normal functioning of the pancreas and carbohydrate metabolism also requires manganese. It plays an important role in the formation of thyroxin, a hormone secreted by the thyroid gland. People with manganese deficiency show weight loss, dermatitis, disturbance in fat metabolism and glucose tolerance, and loss of muscle strength. The recommended dosage is 5 to 10 mg daily.

## Antioxidant Chemicals

**Alpha Lipoic Acid**: Alpha lipoic acid is found in organ meat, red meat, spinach, Brussels sprouts, and potatoes. It is the only fat- and water-soluble antioxidant. It is easily absorbed and transported across cell membranes and may neutralize free radicals both inside and outside of cells. It has the ability to enhance the antioxidant power of vitamins C and E, plus glutathione, in the body, creating an antioxidant network that provides more protection against damaging free radicals. Alpha lipoic acid has been used successfully for nearly thirty years in Germany to reduce the secondary effects of diabetes, including damage to the retina, cataract formation, nerve and heart damage. It improves the blood flow in nerve tissues and improves glucose utilization in the brain, thus protecting nerve tissue against oxidative damage. It can detoxify tissues of heavy metals, such as excessive iron and copper, and the toxic metals, such as lead, cadmium, and mercury. The recommended dosage is 100 to 200 mg daily.

**Coenzyme Q10**: Coenzyme Q10 (CoQ10) is a substance that can actually penetrate into the mitochondria, and it appears to be a vital catalyst in the creation of the energy that cells need for life. It is an essential component of the metabolic process involved in energy (ATP) production. The highest concentration of CoQ10 in our body is in the heart muscle. Research shows a definite link between CoQ10 deficiency and human heart disease. CoQ10 can profoundly increase cardiac function by enhancing the pumping capacity of the heart that results from an increase in the production of energy in the heart muscle cells. CoQ10 supplements have been shown to reenergize aging tissues and to alleviate the effects of many aging-related process and age-related diseases. It can stimulate immunity. Studies showed that immunoglobulin IgG rose significantly in patients receiving doses of 60 mg of CoQ10 per day after two to three months. CoQ10 is valuable in protecting the heart and the brain. Unfortunately, the body's production of CoQ10 begins to decline around age twenty and is seriously deficient by middle age. The recommended dosage for young people is 60 to 100 mg daily, and for seniors, 100 to 300 mg daily. CoQ10 has virtually no side effects, even at very high doses. It is especially helpful for people who take statin drugs, because statins can deplete CoQ10. This may explain why statins cause muscle cramps and pain.

**Resveratrol**: Resveratrol is a substance found in high concentration in the skin and seeds of the grape, plus red wine. It was first identified in 1996 to be capable of interfering with the progression of cancer by inhibiting cancer cell growth. In animal studies it has been found to prevent or slow down progression of illnesses from cancer to cardiovascular disease, and even to extend the life span. Preliminary human studies have shown a range of benefits, including improved blood flow to the heart, reduced blood pressure, and better control of diabetes. The results of human trials on people with untreated diabetes were impressive: it significantly lowered glucose and insulin levels without the patients changing their diet or taking any other drugs. Researchers also found a significant decrease in lipofuscin, a substance that builds up in aging tissues, such as heart muscle cells, liver cells and nerve cells, and is linked to the decline of various tissue and organ functions. Daily dosage is not yet established.

**Quercetin**: Quercetin is a natural free radical fighter found in onion and garlic. It slows the development of cancer through its protective action against the damage caused by carcinogenic substances and its ability to prevent cancer cell growth. It also has specific benefits to the heart. It prevents platelets from sticking to each other and to artery walls and thus may protect against coronary thrombosis and strokes. Clinical studies have found that quercetin can lower total cholesterol, triglycerides, and LDL levels, while raising the HDL level. Daily dosage is not yet established.

**L-carnitine**: L-carnitine (*L* refers to a natural form of carnitine) is an amino acid-like compound found in all human tissue, with the highest concentration occurring in the adrenal glands and heart muscle. It is a vital antioxidant in the creation of energy that heart muscle cells need for life. It is critical for a strong heart because it helps to expand the blood vessels, making the heart's job easier. L-carnitine and CoQ10 are best used together, because of their overlapping mechanisms of action. Research showed that increased levels of L-carnitine in tissues lead to increased fat burning. When L-carnitine takes fat into the mitochondria, fat is transformed into energy. The recommended dosage is 1,000 to 2,000 mg per day.

**Superoxide Dismutases**: Superoxide dismutases (SODs) are a class of closely related enzymes that catalyze the breakdown of the superoxide anion into oxygen and hydrogen peroxide. The human body, especially in young people, produces a profusion of superoxide dismutase. However, in seniors, the body's production of SOD is greatly reduced. SODs are very powerful, endogenous free radical killers. They are present in almost all cells and in extracellular tissue fluids. In humans, SODs contain metal ion cofactors, which can be copper, zinc, or manganese. The copper and zinc SODs are present in the extracellular tissue fluids, while manganese SODs are present in the mitochondria. The mitochondrial SOD is the most biologically important one. In animal studies, mice lacking this mitochondrial SOD die soon after birth. For elderly people, it is advisable to supplement with some antioxidants that can actually penetrate into the mitochondria, such as CoQ10 and alpha lipoic acid, to ensure that you get proper protection of cells against intracellular free radical attacks. Supplemental SOD is not recommended (although it is sold in many stores), because it can be broken down by digestive juices in the gastro-intestinal tract.

**Glutathione**: Glutathione is a powerful antioxidant. It protects every cell, tissue, and organ in the body. Glutathione protects the body against powerful natural and man-made oxidants. It helps the liver detoxify poisonous chemicals and can deactivate at least thirty cancer-causing carcinogens. Glutathione works synergistically with vitamin C and selenium. It maintains healthy immune functions, helps prevent macular degeneration, and helps protect the integrity of red blood cells. Glutathione is manufactured in the liver by three amino acids: glycine, cysteine, and glutamic acid. Supplemental glutathione is of no use (although it is sold in many stores), because it can be broken down into other substances by digestive juices. However, it is found that L-glutamine greatly enhances the body's production of glutathione and can boost blood levels of glutathione. The recommended dosage for L-glutamine is 1,000 mg daily—make sure that you take it with vitamin C and selenium.

## Antioxidant Hormones

**Melatonin**: Melatonin is a hormone produced in the pineal gland, made from the amino acid tryptophan, an essential amino acid that our body does not produce. The body converts tryptophan into the neurotransmitter serotonin, and then at night serotonin is converted into melatonin. Russell Reiter, PhD, who has been researching melatonin for more than thirty years, has concluded that melatonin is the most powerful antioxidant molecule yet to be discovered; it can possibly reset the body's aging clock, turning back the ravages of time. The initial clinical studies on melatonin focused on problems related to the sleep-wake cycle. But today melatonin ranks as one of the important hormones, which stimulates the release of a wide variety of other hormones from the pituitary gland. However, in aging individuals, decreased levels of melatonin are often insufficient to stimulate the release of other hormones (including human growth hormone) in enough quantity to produce health benefits.

Studies have shown that melatonin can boost the immune system by strengthening antibody response, increasing immune cell activity, and moderating the effects of corticosteroid overproduction in response to stress. Melatonin also protects against a variety of neurodegenerative diseases, such as Parkinson's disease, schizophrenia, depression, and Alzheimer's disease. It can also help lower cholesterol, prevent the formation of plaque deposits, and normalize blood pressure.

Recent research has shown that melatonin combats cancer in different ways. It strengthens the immune system's ability to spot and destroy precancerous dysplastic cells, and it can restrain the effect of hormones that can trigger the growth of certain types of cancer, including breast and prostate cancers. In tissue cultures, melatonin has shown to exert a direct, lethal action on estrogen-sensitive breast cancer cells and melanoma cancer cells.

The recommended dosage is 1 to 5 mg daily, depending on age. Hormones are extremely potent biological compounds that are usually effective in small doses. Although melatonin is harmless to the body and causes no side effects other than a natural drowsiness, too much of this hormone causes disuse atrophy of the pineal body. It is important that melatonin only be taken at night, about a half to one hour before bed time. Melatonin is not recommended for people under forty years of age, to avoid interfering with the body's production of the hormone at an early age.

**DHEA**: DHEA (dehydroepiandrosterone) is a naturally occurring steroid derived from another hormone, pregnenolone. It is also produced by the adrenal glands and the brain. DHEA is, in turn, converted into estrogen and testosterone in both women and men. It can stimulate the production of progesterone, cortisone, and the many other steroid hormones as the body needs them.

DHEA is an antiaging nutrient and antioxidant. DHEA appears in the bloodstream at about age seven and then peaks at about age twenty-five. The secretion of this hormone markedly declines with age, and by age seventy it has diminished by 80 to 90 percent. DHEA seems to rejuvenate the systems required for optimal functioning. It appears to reverse many aspects of aging previously thought to be irreversible by correcting much of the deterioration of organs and body systems. Some animal studies have shown great promise for extending the life span. In human trials, some elderly people who suffer from weakness, trembling, muscle wasting, and other signs of aging experience noticeable improvements within several weeks of beginning small doses of DHEA. It has been proven to energize the body, improve memory, lower blood cholesterol, fight obesity, and strengthen the immune system. Several studies have shown that DHEA has a direct and profound effect on the brain's ability to process and store information, and those results have led researchers to believe that DHEA may play a role in preventing Alzheimer's disease (McFarland, J.L., *Aging without Growing Old*. Siloam, 2004).

*The Lancet* reported a study that followed 5,000 women. It found that those who developed breast cancer had lower than average levels of DHEA in their urine as early as nine years before the development of cancer. It is believed that DHEA can block the promotion of carcinogens. In animal experiments, when rats were given an injection of DHEA before introducing the carcinogen, they remained cancer-free. It also increased the life span of these rats by 50 percent.

A long-term study of 242 men between 50 and 79 years of age found that those with the highest levels of DHEA in their blood were only half as likely to die of heart disease as those with relatively little of the hormone (*New England Journal of Medicine*, 315:1519–1524, 1986). After three months of taking DHEA, postmenopausal women showed an 8 to 10 percent decline in total cholesterol levels. Other studies showed a significant decline in patients' propensity to form blood clots.

DHEA appears to protect against both heart disease and stroke. In the Rancho Bernardo study (conducted in Rancho Bernardo, California), researchers found that over a twelve-year period, men with high levels of naturally occurring DHEA had a 40 percent lower risk of heart disease. However, in the follow-up study that covered nineteen years, the risk was only 14 percent lower for those with an elevated DHEA level.

The recommended dosage is 15 to 25 mg per day. The only side effect with doses greater than 90 mg per day is mild masculinization of women, because some of the DHEA is metabolized to testosterone. This side effect goes away when the dosage of DHEA is reduced. The initial studies of DHEA sound very promising and have received a lot of attention in the media and among the public. However, DHEA is a steroid, which can make you feel great for the short term, but over the long term, it may also do some harm to your body, so future research is still needed (Roizen, M., *The Real Age Makeover*. Collins 2004).

DHEA is the precursor to androgens, and high levels of androgens have been linked to prostate cancer in men. A study at Johns Hopkins Medical School found that women who had high levels of male hormones (androgens) had higher incidences of ovarian cancer. Therefore, DHEA should not be taken by men whose laboratory tests show a suspicion of prostate cancer. Women with precancerous dysplastic conditions or suspicion of cancer of reproductive organs should not use DHEA. DHEA also should not be taken by any person who is under forty, pregnant, nursing, or taking any prescription medication. If you decide to take DHEA, you need a complete physical, including measurement of your current DHEA levels. You will also need screenings every six months for prostate cancer as well as measurement of your DHEA levels to make sure they are in the right range.

Antioxidants can protect your body from free radical attacks, both intracellular and extracellular; but some of them may have adverse side effects or even be harmful to your body. Antioxidants, like many substances in our bodies, such as cholesterol, can work both for and against us. Understand their properties and make sure that you know how to use them properly before you decide to take antioxidant supplements. Wise use of antioxidants is important, and one should not be influenced by "high-pressure" marketing and vigorous promotions by supplement-manufacturing companies.

# Chapter 6
# Cardiovascular Disease Is Preventable:
# Have We Missed Doing Something Important?

Cardiovascular disease, the underlying cause of heart attacks and strokes, remains America's leading cause of death. In the United States, 1.5 million people will suffer a heart attack this year, and 300,000 of them will die before they receive medical attention. The estimated number of people in this country living with cardiovascular disease is staggering—12.4 million have coronary heart disease; 4.5 million have had a stroke; and 4.7 million have congestive heart failure. An additional 50 million have high blood pressure.

The total cost to the economy of all that illness is estimated by the American Heart Association at more than $298 billion a year in medical expenses and lost productivity. In spite of the fact that most Americans are aware that prevention and even reversal of some of the common forms of heart disease are possible with changes of lifestyle and diet, heart disease remains the major killer of men and women in this country. Heart disease is generally considered to be preventable.

Have we missed doing something important, or is it simply that not enough of us are listening?

## Understanding Cholesterol and Triglycerides

Cholesterol is a fat-like substance that is absolutely essential to our good health and is necessary for our bodies to function normally. It is used in the body as a building block for our hormones and many complex chemicals. Every cell in the body requires cholesterol. The human body makes 80 percent of its cholesterol from fats, protein, and certain carbohydrates, mainly within the liver. The remaining 20 percent comes from dietary sources. A balancing mechanism exists so that there is always enough cholesterol for the cells to function properly: the more you eat, the less your body makes, and vice versa. Unfortunately, this mechanism ensures a sufficient supply of cholesterol inside the cells without regards to levels circulating in the blood. When blood cholesterol level rises above a certain level, the excess is converted into bile and excreted into the duodenum through the common bile duct. Human bodies synthesize about 3,000 to 4,000 mg of cholesterol per day and receive only a small amount in their food, mainly from eggs and animal fat.

The body uses cholesterol to manufacture vital hormones, including pituitary hormones, adrenal hormones, DHEA, pregnenolone, aldosterone, testosterone, and estrogen. The adrenal glands contain the highest concentration of cholesterol of any tissue in the body in order to synthesize adrenal hormones. The brain and spinal cord account for only 2 percent of total body weight, and yet they contain almost one fourth of the total cholesterol in the body. The brain uses cholesterol to make neurotransmitters that conduct nerve impulses throughout the body. Cholesterol is a critical structural support in cell membranes and also an important building block of the insulation around nerves, which ensures that nerve impulses are conducted appropriately.

Since 1950, researchers have found that people with high blood levels of a type of fat-protein combination called high-density lipoproteins (HDLs, the so-called "good" cholesterol) did not have heart attacks; in contrast, people with high levels of another kind of fat-protein combination called low-density lipoproteins (LDLs, the so-called "bad" cholesterol) were at high risk of having heart attacks. The density is based on the weight of the lipoprotein molecule: HDLs are high in protein and low in cholesterol, and LDLs have little protein and high levels of cholesterol. It is postulated that HDL cholesterol carries cholesterol from the arterial wall to the liver, where it is recycled for further use or excreted into the duodenum through the common bile duct; LDL cholesterol moves through the arteries and tends to leave accumulations of cholesterol in the blood vessel walls, leading to atherosclerosis and heart attacks. Therefore, the higher the HDL level, the lower the risk of heart attacks. The desirable ratio of LDLs to HDLs is less than 3.5; as the ratio rises, so does the risk.

Triglycerides are glycerol molecules attached to three fatty acids; they serve the body both as the primary storage form of fat and as a basic fuel for muscle tissue. They are produced in the process of converting excess carbohydrates into stored body fat and are linked to heart disease. Blood triglyceride levels increase when you eat refined carbohydrates: products made with white sugar, anything made with white flour, and even sweetened fruit juices. Diets high in complex carbohydrates, such as whole grains, vegetables, and seeds, do not have the same effect. Obesity is probably the major cause of elevated triglycerides. Other situations that can lead to high triglyceride levels include alcohol abuse and the use of certain drugs, some diuretics, oral contraceptives, and products containing female hormones. Triglycerides are also important in determining heart disease risk. New studies show that people with high triglyceride levels and a low level of HDL cholesterol increase the risk of heart disease. A ratio of triglycerides divided by the HDL that exceeds 5.5 indicates heart disease risk; as the number climbs, so does the risk.

Saturated fats found primarily in animal foods and dairy products raise blood cholesterol by slowing the removal of LDL cholesterol from the blood. This is the reason you may develop high blood cholesterol levels even if your diet is low in cholesterol but high in saturated fat. Polyunsaturated and monounsaturated fats lower LDL cholesterol in the blood when substituted for saturated fats in the diet. (Be aware that when vegetable oils are converted into margarine by hydrogenation to make it firm, it becomes more saturated, strongly proinflammatory, and increases extra heart disease risk.)

Here are the currently established numbers regarding blood cholesterol levels for assessing the risk of heart disease:

A.  Total cholesterol levels

 1.   200 mg/dl or less: desirable

 2.   200–239 mg/dl: borderline

 3.   240 mg/dl and higher: too high

B.  LDL cholesterol levels

 1.   130 mg/dl or less: desirable

 2.   130–159 mg/dl: borderline

 3.   160 mg/dl and higher: too high

C.  HDL cholesterol levels for men

 1.   45 mg/dl: desirable

 2.   35–45 mg/dl: borderline

 3.   35 mg/dl and lower: too low

D.  HDL cholesterol levels for women

1. 55 mg/dl: desirable

2. 40–55 mg/dl: borderline

3. 40 mg/dl and lower: too low

E. Triglyceride levels

1. 200 mg/dl: desirable

2. 200–400 mg/dl: borderline

3. 400–1000 mg/dl: high

4. 1,000 mg/dl and higher: very high

## Mechanism of Atherosclerosis

In atherosclerosis, the inner layers of artery walls of the larger arteries and those that supply the heart, called coronary arteries, become thick and irregular. Many macrophages congregate in the artery lining, where they trap oxidized LDL cholesterol. This causes the formation of foam cells (macrophages containing fat have a foamy appearance) that coalesce into fatty streaks. Upon combining with calcium deposits, they form scab-like plaque on the artery lining. These plaques have the potential to rupture and further clog or obstruct the arteries. Over time, this gradual buildup eventually infiltrates the artery wall. This process narrows the channel and reduces the blood supply to the affected area, increasing the risks of heart attacks, stroke, and other serious arterial diseases.

In most heart attacks, a blood clot forms in a plaque rupture site, suddenly blocking blood flow. The location of the obstruction and duration of reduced blood flow determine the extent of damage and complications. Sometimes part or all of an atherosclerotic plaque in the systemic artery breaks off and travels through the blood to distant sites. The moving blood clot, an embolus, may lodge in the brain, legs, kidneys, or intestine, and is potentially life-threatening.

Inflammation is the process by which our body responds to an infection or injury. Researchers have suggested that inflammation is also an important factor in atherosclerosis. The major injurious factors that promote atherogenesis (the production of atherosclerotic plaques), including cigarette smoking, hypertension, and hyperglycemia, are well established. Inflammation is thought to contribute not only to the formation of plaque but may also contribute to its disruption, resulting in the formation of a blood clot. These correlations seem to be consistent with pathological examinations of the artery walls of people with atherosclerosis, which show that inflammation is virtually always a component.

It appears that coronary heart disease and atherosclerosis begin as an inflammatory process in the lining of arteries. C-reactive protein (CRP) is one of the acute phase proteins that increase during systemic inflammation. A more sensitive CRP test, a highly sensitive C-reactive protein (hs-CRP) assay, is now being considered as an additional test to assess cardiovascular disease risk. The American Heart Association and the Centers for Disease Control and Prevention released a joint statement in 2003 on the use of inflammatory markers in clinical and public health practice. This statement was developed after reviewing the evidence of that association between inflammatory markers such as CRP and coronary heart disease and stroke.

Clinical studies have found that high levels of hs-CRP consistently predict recurrent coronary diseases in patients with unstable angina and acute myocardial infarction. Higher hs-CRP levels are associated with lower survival rates and may increase the risk that an artery will reclose after it's been opened by balloon angioplasty. High levels of hs-CRP in the blood may also predict prognosis and recurrent events in patients with stroke and peripheral arterial disease.

The currently used numbers of hs-CRP levels for a person with a low risk of developing cardiovascular disease is less than 1.0 mg/L. If hs-CPR is 1.0 to 3.0 mg/L, a person has an average risk. If hs-CRP is higher than 3.0 mg/L, a person is at high risk. However, patients with infectious diseases, autoimmune diseases, or cancer may also have elevated hs-CRP levels. Therefore, if a patient exhibits persistent and markedly elevated hs-CRP (higher than 10.0 mg/L), non-cardiovascular causes should be excluded.

Researchers have also found that a high level of blood serum homocysteine is a powerful risk factor for cardiovascular disease, because homocysteine is a corrosive amino acid that can damage endothelial cells, the inner lining cells of artery walls, promoting atherosclerosis and blood clot formation. Homocysteine is not obtained directly from the diet but is strongly influenced by an animal protein-rich diet, especially in people with deficiencies of vitamin B-12 and folic acid. It is produced as a byproduct of the metabolism of methionine, an essential amino acid abundant after meat digestion. Normally, it is further converted into cysteine with the aid of vitamin B-12 and folic acid. It is the inefficient conversion of homocysteine into cysteine due to deficiencies of vitamin B-12 and folic acid that allow a high level of homocysteine to accumulate in the bloodstream. Homocysteine blood serum levels higher than 11.4 µmol/L for men and higher than 10.4 µmol/L for women indicate high risk.

## How Much Can Cholesterol-Lowering Drugs Reduce Risk of Cardiovascular Disease?

For the time being, the first line of therapy to reduce risk for cardiovascular disease is to change your diet and lifestyle. If blood cholesterol levels fail to respond adequately, expect medications to be recommended by your doctor. The best-known treatment, the use of cholesterol-lowering drugs called statins, remains the most common. Such drugs are the best-selling medicines in history, used by more than thirteen million Americans and an additional twelve million patients around the world, producing $27.8 billion in sales in 2006. Since a high cholesterol level is just one of the risk factors for coronary heart disease, how much can cholesterol-lowering drugs actually reduce risks of cardiovascular disease? This is the question frequently asked in recent years.

In fact, the cholesterol levels of many patients with heart disease are not much higher than those without heart disease. The Framingham Study reported that half of the people who died of heart attacks did not have high blood cholesterol levels. Researchers suggest that, except among high-risk heart patients, the benefits of statins such as Lipitor can be overstated. James Wright, MD, a professor at the University of British Columbia, found no benefit in people over the age of sixty-five, no matter how much their cholesterol was reduced, and also no benefit in women of any age; although he did observe a small reduction in the number of heart attacks for middle-aged men taking statins in clinical trials. For these middle-aged men, there was no overall reduction in total deaths, despite big reductions in LDL levels. In his opinion, most people are taking something with no chance of benefit and a risk of harm. As discussed before, cholesterol is necessary for our bodies to function normally and is essential to our good health. There is evidence that low total cholesterol levels (below 180 mg/dl) are associated with a high risk of death in older people and low LDL cholesterol levels (below 80 mg/dl) with a higher risk of bleeding stroke (*Lancet*, August 2001; *Circulation*, April 2009).

If you compare the rate of heart disease in different countries, the claim made regarding the usefulness of cholesterol-lowering drugs by the pharmaceutical companies on prime time television ("cholesterol-lowering drugs reduce the risk of heart attack by 39 to 60 percent") is even more doubtful. The Swiss have higher cholesterol levels than those of Americans, but their rate of heart disease is lower. The Spaniards have LDL levels similar to those of Americans but less than half the rate of heart disease. Australian aborigines have low cholesterol levels but high rate of heart disease. The Greenland's Inuit people get most of their calories from fish, seal blubber, and whale meat. In spite of their high cholesterol intake, they rarely die from heart disease.

All these findings and reports appear to say that there are other contributing factors in the pathogenesis of heart attacks. The cholesterol factor is not the only important factor. The extent of the role that cholesterol-lowering drugs are playing in reducing the risk of cardiovascular disease needs to be readdressed, if we're going to make anymore headway in preventing heart attacks and strokes.

When we review the mechanism of how lipids are absorbed in the body in relation to the formation of plaques in the coronary artery wall, leading to a heart attack, we can clearly see that diets rich in saturated fat, cholesterol, and trans fat affect the coronary arteries with cholesterol deposits before most other arteries in our body. This may explain why more heart attacks in high risk people for coronary disease occur after major holidays, such as Christmas through New Year's, during which time people tend to overindulge in foods, and holiday foods tend to be heavily laden with bad fats. The occurrence of such heart attacks can be totally unrelated to the patients' cholesterol levels before the holiday. This may, perhaps, explain the limits of what cholesterol-lowering drugs can do.

Absorption of lipid nutrients by the intestinal tract is different from that of proteins and carbohydrates. After protein is digested to the molecular level in the intestinal tract, the digested products (amino acid molecules) are absorbed by the villi, which are minute projections of the mucous membrane of the distal small intestines, the jejunum and ileum. They are then transported to the liver through the portal vein. Simple carbohydrates, such as candies, are already more or less at the molecular level, ready to be absorbed into the bloodstream after they pass through the stomach. For complex carbohydrates, the digested products are absorbed and then transported to the liver along much the same pathway as for protein absorption.

However, digested lipid nutrients are absorbed at the molecular level into the central lacteals, which are minute lymph-carrying vessels in the villi. Lipid nutrients are then transported through lymphatic channels into the cisterna chyli, a dilated station formed by the convergence of lymphatic trunks in the abdomen. The lymph in the abdominal lymphatic channels and cisterna chyli usually appears milky white after fatty meals because of the presence of fat globules in the proteinaceous lymph, known as chyle. The fat-containing lymph, or chyle, ascends through the thoracic duct in the posterior mediastinum and ends in the junction of the left subclavian and internal jugular veins, a close distance from the heart. This means that any absorbed saturated fats, trans fats, and cholesterol reach coronary arteries before most other arteries in our body (see diagram). This anatomical distribution is certainly unfavorable for coronary heart disease.

During my practice of medicine, I saw several patients with ruptures of the thoracic duct due to trauma or cancer invasion. The fluids that leaked from the thoracic duct appeared just like milk and were sometimes tinged with blood. Can you imagine how many dietary fats are introduced into your bloodstream after a heavy meal?

The fat-containing lymph is transported directly to the bloodstream and returns to the heart quickly. Any fat in the blood reaches the coronary arteries almost immediately after the blood is pumped out from the heart. Coronary arteries are the first to emerge from the ascending aorta, which is the main trunk of the systemic arteries and carries blood away from the heart. This may explain why statin-type drugs, which exert their cholesterol-lowering action in the liver, can only play a limited role in reducing the risk of cardiovascular disease.

However, reducing your intake of foods containing trans fat, saturated fat, and cholesterol, replacing them with omega-3 fatty acids (especially marine types), and increasing supplementation of lecithin, which acts as a powerful emulsifying agent in the blood to help dissolve cholesterol, may help you lower your blood cholesterol level in a way that will not burden the coronary arteries and does not cause any adverse side effects.

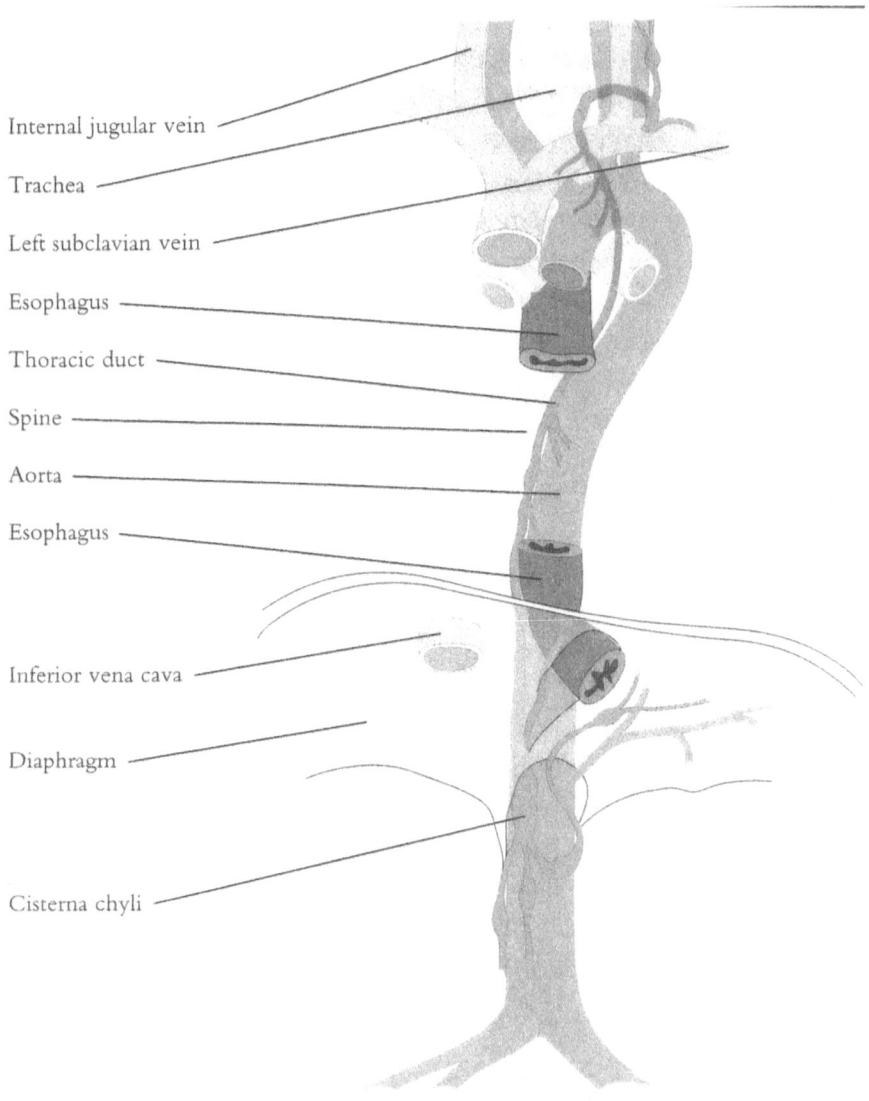

Internal jugular vein

Trachea

Left subclavian vein

Esophagus

Thoracic duct

Spine

Aorta

Esophagus

Inferior vena cava

Diaphragm

Cisterna chyli

Diagram of Lipid Absorption: Lipid nutrients are absorbed into central lacteals in the villi and then transported into the cisterna chyli. The thoracic duct arises in the cistern chyli and returns the chyle and lymph from the entire body below the diaphragm directly to the bloodstream. It ascends through the posterior mediastinum and ends in the junction of the left subclavian and internal jugular veins.

## The Whole-Body Approach to Reducing the Risk of Cardiovascular Disease

The whole-body approach to reducing the risk of cardiovascular disease does not deal with just one or two contributing factors. Instead, it promotes the idea of letting the whole body work together synergistically to protect your heart health in the most efficient way. In the late nineteen nineties, I was at risk for cardiovascular disease, but thanks to this whole-body approach, I am no longer a member of that high-risk group. In retrospect, I feel I am very lucky that moderate to severe hypertension didn't cripple me, and heart attacks didn't recur. I hope that sharing this information is helpful to those who might wish to benefit from my example. The measures taken were as follows:

1. Bring the body back to optimal physiological condition, at a healthy pH of 7.4 in the tissue fluids, using morning fasting saliva pH test as a guide. The increased alkaline reserve in the body can be used to neutralize the acidic products after consuming animal protein. This is especially useful whenever there are "acid tides," when a large amount of strongly acidic products enter the bloodstream after a meal high in animal protein, fat, and sugar, which also increases free radical attacks. The alkaline reserve can immediately neutralize strongly acidic products, such as sulfuric acid, phosphoric acid, uric acid, and amino acids, including corrosive homocysteine. In retrospect, this may have protected me from heart attacks in the past after occasional overindulgences in foods and bad fats.

Suggested Measures

a. Drink a glass of freshly squeezed vegetable and fruit juice (200 to 250 ml) every morning. Choose five or six from the following: celery, onion, cucumber, zucchini, carrot, radish, bitter melon, green apple, green papaya, and pear. The amount of each variety can be adjusted to your taste. Make your own recipe. This measure offers a boost of alkaline reserves and is highly recommended to anyone who wishes to improve his or her cardiovascular health.

b. If your morning fasting saliva pH test indicates an acidic pH, decrease acidifying foods to 20 percent of your diet and increase alkalizing foods to 80 percent every day until the pH of your fasting saliva pH test becomes healthy (7.2 to 7.6). Then you may allow more acidifying foods, up to no more than 30 percent. Use the pH reading from the morning fasting saliva pH test as a guide, and adjust the various portions of acidifying and alkalizing foods in your diet accordingly.

c. When you drink water from the same source for a long period of time, make sure that the water has a pH close to 7.4 and contains the minerals your body needs. If you drink beverages like tea and coffee every day, try not to add sugar and cream, both of which are acidifying. Forget about carbonated soft drinks, especially those containing phosphates and a large amount of sugar, which are strongly acidifying and unhealthy.

d. The benefits of regular exercise to the cardiovascular system are well documented. Prolonged periods of inactivity can affect the body's ability to process fats and other substances that contribute to heart disease risk. Furthermore, regular exercise also helps contribute to the proper pH level in the tissue fluids. By increasing the excretion of acidic waste through perspiration and by increasing carbon dioxide output through expiration, regular exercise can tilt the pH of tissue fluids toward alkalinity.

2. Boost the immune system to restrain the inflammatory response in tissues. Inflammatory process is known to be involved in

every aspect of atherosclerosis. It contributes not only to the formation of plaque but may also contribute to its disruption, resulting in the formation of a blood clot. If your daily diet contains excessive proinflammatory foods, such as trans fats, your risk for cardiovascular disease increases.

Suggested Measures

a. A proper diet with necessary supplements is essential for a healthy immune system. Our immune system needs thirteen kinds of vitamins, sixteen essential minerals and trace elements, eight essential amino acids, and two essential fatty acids to function optimally. In addition to proper diet, take a multivitamin pill and omega-3 fish oil soft gels daily. As discussed before, EPA omega-3 fatty acids can reduce blood clotting and restrain the inflammatory response in tissues. A thousand milligrams of omega-3 fish oil is recommended every day. If you belong to the high-risk group, increase the level to 2,000 mg of omega-3 fish oil every day. According to the American Heart Association, consuming omega-3 fatty acids in fish or supplements significantly reduces subsequent cardiac and all-cause mortality, further confirmed by a recent finding discussed in chapter 10.

b. Folic acid (400 to 800 mcg daily) together with vitamin B-12 (500 to 1,000 mcg daily) are highly recommended in order to maintain normal blood serum levels of homocysteine.

At least 400 mg of magnesium a day is also recommended for those at high risk for coronary disease. A ten-year study on 400 people at high risk for coronary disease found that those who ate a magnesium rich diet had less than half as many complications from cardiovascular-related problems as those who ate only about one-third of the amount of magnesium. You should eliminate all pro-inflammatory foods, such as margarine, lard, and hardened, processed, man-made fat, from your diet.

    c.   Lecithin is an essential constituent of all living cells of the human body. It forms 30 percent of the dry weight of the brain and 73 percent of the total liver fat. All atherosclerosis is characterized by an increase of blood cholesterol and a decrease in lecithin. Lecithin acts as a powerful emulsifying agent in the blood to help dissolve cholesterol. HDL cholesterol is manufactured partly from the body's natural emulsifier, lecithin. The primary role of lecithin in cardiovascular health is its ability to lower the cholesterol level. The arteries are protected from fatty buildup when lecithin is added to the diet. Daily addition of one or two tablespoons of granular lecithin, mixed with your cereal or drink, or 2,400 to 3,600 mg of soft gels helps protect your cardiovascular health.

    d.   Reduce stress. Stress suppresses your immune system and decreases the ability in tissues, including arterial walls, to contain the inflammatory response. Stress-reduction measures, such as aerobic exercise, yoga, and tai chi, plus some form of relaxation, such as hobbies, a massage, listening to music, and meditation, can be tried as a first step to gaining control. Individual stress management consultations or programs are offered by some hospitals and medical schools.

3.  Controlling free radical attacks to reduce oxidative reactions is another measure to reduce the risk of cardiovascular disease. This is especially important for seniors, because the production of superoxide dismutase, a powerful, endogenous free radical killer, is greatly decreased with advancing age. In heart disease, free radicals promote the oxidation of LDL, which tends to

accumulate as fatty plaques in the artery walls. Hardened fats should be avoided, because they increase the amount of oxidation in the body, resulting in greater numbers of free radicals roaming in your body. Antioxidants that are beneficial in protecting our cardiovascular health include vitamin C, vitamin E, beta-carotene, CoQ10, quercetin, resveratrol, and L-carnitine.

Suggested Measures

a. Wise use of antioxidants: Several antioxidants provide beneficial effects on the health of the cardiovascular system.

*Vitamin C decreases total cholesterol, LDL, and triglycerides, and it increases good HDL. British and Swedish scientists have reported that vitamin C reduces blood platelet adhesion by reducing the stickiness of the blood. German researchers found that 1,000 mg daily of vitamin C normalized blood platelet adhesion and reduced the interaction of platelets within the arterial walls.

*Vitamin E helps dissolve fresh clots and prevents their formation in arteries and veins and helps prevent arterial and venous thrombosis, or clots, in the circulatory system of the brain. Vitamin E acts as a surfactant, so it minimizes the tendency of blood platelets to stick together and form clots. A significant decrease in adhesiveness of platelets was noted after two weeks of daily supplementation with 400 IU of vitamin E. The Cambridge Heart Antioxidant Study found a 75 percent reduction in new heart attacks in the vitamin E group compared to the placebo group. Beta-carotene benefits the heart with many of the same antioxidant reasons as vitamin E.

*CoQ10 is involved in energy (ATP) production in our body. The highest concentration of CoQ10 in our body is in the heart muscle. Researchers have found a definite link between CoQ10 deficiency and heart disease. CoQ10 can profoundly increase cardiac function by enhancing the pumping capacity of the heart, resulting from an increase in the production of energy in heart muscle cells. It is especially helpful for people who take statin drugs, because statins can deplete CoQ10. This may explain why statins cause muscle cramps and pain.

*Quercetin prevents platelets from sticking to each other and to artery walls and may protect against coronary thrombosis and strokes. Clinical studies show that quercetin can lower total cholesterol, triglycerides, and LDL levels, while raising HDL levels.

*Resveratrol is found primarily in the skin and seeds of the grape. One liter of red wine contains up to two grams of resveratrol, which was first identified in 1996 as being capable of interfering with the progression of cancer by inhibiting cancer cell growth. Preliminary human studies have shown benefits of improving blood flow to the heart, lowering blood pressure, and reducing risk factors for heart disease.

* L-carnitine is a vital antioxidant in the creation of energy that heart muscle cells need for life. It is critical for a strong heart because it helps to expand the blood vessels, making the heart's job easier. Research showed that increased levels of L-carnitine in tissues lead to increased fat burning, and thus fat was transformed into energy.

b.  Here's a special heart health-promoting recipe.

## Red Wine with Onion

One large onion, cut into small pieces

Soak the onion in 750 ml of red wine for ten days.

Strain, and discard the onion before drinking the wine, 100 ml per day.

This do-it-yourself, "enhanced" red wine recipe is my strategy for protection against cardiovascular disease and cancer. Researchers have found that alcohol at low doses is beneficial, and this benefit appears more pronounced in wine (especially red wine) drinkers, based on the analysis of mortality rates related to cardiovascular disease and cancer in eighteen countries. The moderate ethanol intake causes an increase in HDL blood levels and a decrease in the tendency of blood to form clots by inhibiting blood platelet aggregation. A Danish study showed that moderate wine consumption induced a 40 percent decrease in the risk of death related to cardiovascular disease and a 22 percent decrease in cancer mortality risk. Coincidentally, onion offers similar specific benefits to the heart, plus an ability to prevent cancer cell growth. They seem to have overlapping mechanisms of action, and their combination offers inevitably better results. Furthermore, the health-promoting ingredient quercetin in the onion is very water soluble and can be easily eliminated through rinsing the peeled bulb under running water and cooking. If the onion is soaked in red wine, the quercetin is fully preserved and further enhances the valuable effects of red wine. After ten days of soaking, the unpleasant, pungent flavor of raw onion is practically gone. As a matter of fact, I have been consuming this "enhanced" red wine for several years, and I really enjoy it.

c. Pure pomegranate juice (4 to 8 oz per day) is a highly recommended addition to your breakfast menu. In recent years it has become the antioxidant of choice for people at high risk for cardiovascular disease; as it is very rich in polyphenols; it also demonstrates a high capacity for scavenging free radicals. It has been shown to inhibit LDL oxidation and to arrest atherosclerosis development both in vitro and in vivo. Researchers have also found that pomegranate juice (8 oz/day) improved blood flow to the heart by 17 percent after 3 months and decreased arterial plaques by 30 percent after one year. Other studies showed that daily consumption of pomegranate juice could reduce carotid artery stenosis, LDL oxidation, and blood pressure (*Clinical Nutrition* 23:423-33, 2004).

There is a great deal we can do naturally and nutritionally to enhance the health of the heart and to prevent instances of cardiovascular disease. First, bring your body back to optimal physiological condition, with a healthy pH of 7.4 in tissue fluids. Then the body's increased alkaline reserve can neutralize the acidic products resulting from animal protein digestion and stabilize the acid-alkaline balance in the tissue fluids. Second, boost the immune system, so it can restrain the inflammatory response in tissues, including artery walls where atherosclerotic plaque is formed. Third, strictly control free radical attacks. In that way, we can reduce oxidative reactions, including oxidation of LDL, and thus reduce the formation of fatty plaque. This whole-body approach to reducing the risk of cardiovascular disease is intended to allow the whole body to work together synergistically to protect your heart health and increase the chance of success. We cannot depend on any one measure or one drug to ward off cardiovascular disease.

# Chapter 7
# Osteoporosis Can Be Prevented and Reversed

Osteoporosis causes 1.5 million fractures a year in the United States, making it the nation's leading cause of broken bones. These fractures include 700,000 vertebral and 300,000 hip fractures, which are often life-threatening. During the year after a hip fracture, 25 percent of patients die, and one-third of patients who break a hip due to osteoporosis never regain their independence.

Currently eight million American women over age fifty have osteoporosis. Another thirty-four million have osteopenia, which is lower than optimal bone mineral density. The National Osteoporosis Foundation estimates that at least two million men currently have osteoporosis, and millions more could be at risk. According to the National Institute of Arthritis and Musculoskeletal and Skin Diseases, about 6 percent of all men over fifty will experience a hip fracture and about 5 percent will fracture a spinal bone as a result of osteoporosis. A 2008 article in the *New England Journal of Medicine* suggested that osteoporosis in men is underdiagnosed and undertreated. In fact, hip fractures are more serious for men than women. Men are more likely than women to die within a year of breaking a hip bone (*New England Journal of Medicine*, August 2008).

Osteoporotic fractures result in 800,000 emergency room visits, 500,000 hospitalizations, and 2.6 million doctor visits annually. In 2002, medical care for osteoporotic fractures alone cost $18 billion. As a result, the US government has declared 2002 through 2012 as the National Bone and Joint Disease Decade.

## Understanding Osteoporosis

The underlying mechanism in all cases of osteoporosis is an imbalance between bone formation and bone resorption. In normal bone, there is constant bone matrix remodeling at any point in time throughout a person's life. Bone is resorbed by osteoclasts, after which new bone is deposited by osteoblasts. Osteoblasts and osteoclasts are coupled together; the purpose is to regulate calcium homeostasis, repair micro-damage, and also to shape and sculpt the skeleton during growth.

Bones serve as reserves for important minerals, most notably calcium and phosphorus, and buffer the blood against excessive pH changes by absorbing or releasing alkaline salts. During bone resorption by the osteoclasts, the stored calcium is released into the systemic circulation. During bone formation, circulating calcium in its mineral form is removed from the bloodstream. This is an import process in regulating calcium balance.

The main mechanism by which osteoporosis develops is inadequate bone mass during growth when excessive bone resorption is accompanied by inadequate formation of new bone during remodeling.

Calcium metabolism plays a significant role in bone turnover. When deficiencies of calcium and vitamin D leads to impaired bone deposition, and also in situations when the blood pH needs to be adjusted to maintain its physiologically optimal pH of 7.4, alkaline calcium compounds, such as calcium carbonate, are leached from the bones to ensure sufficient calcium in the blood and to restore the acid-alkaline balance to the optimal pH of 7.4.

At the present time, the highest rates of osteoporotic hip fractures are noted among North Americans, Australians, northern Europeans, and New Zealanders. Hip fracture is much less of a problem in Asia, South America, and Africa. The countries that consume the most calcium appear to have the highest rates of osteoporotic fractures, and studies in those countries have also showed that milk (fortified with calcium), dairy foods, and additional calcium (800 to 1,200 mg/day) by themselves or in any combination do not prevent osteoporotic fractures among many people (Lanou, A.J. and Castleman, M., *Building Bone Vitality.* McGraw-Hill, 2009). It becomes clear that there are other contributing factors also involved in calcium metabolism, which pulls calcium out of the bloodstream into the bone or vice versa.

Osteoporosis itself has no specific symptoms; its main consequence is the increased risk of bone fractures. When fractures occur in situations where healthy people would not normally break a bone, it is a sign of osteoporosis. If bone loss is occurring, a few signs suggestive of osteoporosis warrant further investigation. These signs include frequent nighttime leg cramps, heavy plaque formation around the teeth, periodontal disease, receding gums, recurrent kidney stone formation, and frequent lower back pain. Osteoporotic fractures usually occur in the vertebral column, hip, rib, and wrist. Osteoporosis is defined as having a bone mineral density T score of minus 2.5 or lower. Lesser degrees of bone loss are known as osteopenia.

**Primary Causes of Development of Osteoporosis**

As discussed before, in any normal bone in our body, there is a constant matrix remodeling of the bone. Up to 10 percent of all bone mass may be undergoing remodeling at any point in time. The bone is resorbed by osteoclasts, after which new bone is deposited by osteoblasts; this process takes place continually during our entire life.

Bone acts as reserves for minerals, most notably calcium and phosphorus. Calcium is involved in many bodily activities, including blood clotting, cell division, maintenance of immune function, and the production of energy. Calcium is also crucial for nerve conduction and muscle contraction. If our diet becomes low in calcium, the body begins taking calcium from our bones to compensate for this deficiency, thinning them and making them brittle in the process, leading to osteoporosis.

Levels of calcium and phosphorus in the diet play an important role in controlling bone loss. As the diet becomes higher in phosphorus and lower in calcium, bone breakdown and calcium loss from the bone increases through the secretion of parathyroid hormone. The calcium-phosphorus ratio (10:4) in the blood must stay constant even at the expense of your bones, so the intake of calcium and phosphorus should be approximately equal. If the diet is equal in calcium and phosphorus, the blood calcium will be at the optimal proportion of two and a half times higher than phosphorus. In fact, mother's milk has the same calcium-phosphorus ratio as in the blood.

The average American diet is very high in phosphorus in relation to calcium. Here are a few examples of the calcium-phosphorus ratios in 100 g of common foods (from the US government *Composition of Foods Handbook*):

1. Beef and most red meat—11 mg:207 mg

2. Cottage cheese—94 mg:152 mg

3. Milk—118 mg:93 mg

4. Wheat bran—119 mg:1,276 mg

5. Rice bran—76 mg:1,386 mg

6. Wheat germ—72 mg:1,118 mg

7. Wheat flour—45 mg:423 mg

8. Oatmeal—21 mg:138 mg

9. Dark greens (broccoli, kale, watercress and collard)—184 mg:37 mg

In addition, one 8-oz can of a carbonated soft drink contains 136 mg of phosphorus, with no calcium. We have become more dependent upon highly processed foods, which are also low in calcium and high in phosphorus. This is one reason why we need to take a calcium supplement. French researchers reported that among elderly women who completed eighteen months of daily supplementation with 1,000 mg of calcium and 800 IU of vitamin D, the number of hip fractures was 43 percent lower and the total number of nonvertebral fractures was 32 percent lower, compared with those receiving a placebo (*New England Journal of Medicine*, December 1992). However, other studies show that daily supplementation with calcium and vitamin D does not prevent hip fractures in some people. It appears that there are other contributing factors involved in the mechanism of developing osteoporosis, and daily supplementation with calcium and vitamin D alone does not guarantee protection in those people (*The New York Times*, Personal Health. November 24, 2009).

Bone contains three calcium compounds: calcium carbonate, hydroxide, and phosphate. When the blood pH falls below pH 7.4, the body must correct it as quickly as possible by pulling alkaline calcium compounds from the bone into the blood to neutralize the excess acids. Harvard researchers found that high consumption of animal protein was associated with an increased risk of osteoporotic fractures *(American Journal of Public Health*, 87:992, 1997). Animal protein after digestion in the intestinal tract is broken down into twenty-two component amino acids that are absorbed and transported to the liver through the portal vein. The amino acids are synthesized into various kinds of protein, according to the body's needs.

The problem arises when the protein in your diet exceeds what your body needs. Because there is no storage for excess protein, superfluous amino acids are processed into ammonia in the kidneys, and the liver quickly converts ammonia into urea, producing endogenous acid products in the body. If this occurs persistently, these acid products lower the pH of the blood and tissue fluids and trigger the homeostatic cycle of pulling alkaline calcium compounds from the bone into the bloodstream to neutralize the excess acids. During this process, more calcium tends to be drawn into the blood than the situation requires. The kidneys retain this excess calcium from the blood and return part of it to the bloodstream; and the rest is excreted in urine.

As the amount of protein in the diet increases, so does the amount of calcium excreted in urine. According to the National Academy of Sciences, 1 g of dietary protein increases urinary calcium excretion by 1 to 1.5 mg. So if your diet contains about 20 g of excess protein (far more than your body needs), you lose 20 to 30 mg of calcium. Toronto researchers fed adult participants two different diets containing the same number of calories but different amounts of protein for one month. On the high-protein diet, participants' daily urinary calcium output increased 63 percent (*International Journal of Epidemiology*, 21:953, 1992). British researchers reported that people who ate the most meat, fish, eggs, and grains and the fewest fruits and vegetables had the lowest bone mineral density (BMD). As their fruit and vegetable consumption increased relative to animal foods, their BMD also increased (Lanou, A.J. and Castleman, M., *Building Bone Vitality*. McGraw-Hill, 2009).

In one recent study, 171 healthy men and women were treated with either alkaline bicarbonate (equivalent to nine servings of fruits and vegetables daily) or no bicarbonate. The former group experienced much lower levels of calcium loss, as well as loss of N-telopeptide, the biochemical marker of bone resorption, in the urine. Researchers concluded that increasing the alkaline content of the diet by eating more fruits and vegetables can be a safe and low-cost approach to preventing osteoporosis (*Journal of Clinical Endocrinology and Metabolism*, January 2009). It's clear that a constant, high-protein diet that increases urinary calcium loss and weakens bones is another significant risk factor for osteoporosis.

## The Whole-Body Approach to Reducing the Risk of Osteoporosis

Currently, prevention of bone fracture is the focus in treating osteoporosis. To minimize the likelihood of bone fractures, present efforts zero in on the preservation of bone mass in people with normal bone density or improvement of bone mass in people with low bone density. It seems that these measures make sense. However, there is growing controversy about osteoporosis drugs. There are many reports of low-trauma fractures of the thigh bone or other major bones occurring even though these drugs are supposed to prevent them. At the 2010 annual meeting of the American Academy of Orthopedic Surgeons, researchers presented data suggesting that after four or five years of treatment with these drugs, some bone may lose its structural integrity and become brittle.

The whole-body approach makes use of every aspect of antiosteoporotic measures to obtain a balance between bone resorption and bone formation.

1.  Bring your body back to optimal physiological condition with a healthy pH of 7.4 in your tissue fluids, using morning fasting saliva pH tests as a guide, so as to increase the alkaline reserve in the tissue fluids of your body. Adequate alkaline reserves can neutralize the acid produced after consuming animal protein, stabilizing the acid-alkaline balance in the tissue fluids and the blood and thus preventing the need to pull calcium compounds from the bone.

Suggested Measures

a.   Have a glass of freshly squeezed vegetable and fruit juice (200 to 250 ml) every morning. Choose five or six of the following: celery, onion, cucumber, zucchini, carrot, radish, bitter melon, green apple, green papaya, and pear. The amount of each variety can be adjusted to your taste. Make your own recipe. This measure is highly recommended for those who are at risk for osteoporosis, because it efficiently boosts your alkaline reserve in the tissue fluids.

b.   If you have osteopenia, eat 20 percent acidifying foods and 80 percent alkalizing foods at each meal. You can make use of the pH results of your morning fasting saliva pH test as a guide to adjust the various portions of acidifying and alkalizing foods. Do not consume more protein than your body needs.

c.   Make sure that the water you drink every day, if it is from one source, has a pH close to 7.4 and contains the minerals your body needs. Boil tap water to get rid of chlorine before you test or drink it. When you drink tea and coffee, which are alkalizing beverages, preferably do not add sugar and cream, both of which are acidifying. Forget about carbonated soft drinks, which are acidifying.

d.   Participate in physical exercise. Weight-bearing exercises are the most important things we can do to keep our bones strong. Regular exercise improves energy levels, enhances blood circulation, and increases the appetite, thus furthering the nourishment of cells, including osteoblasts and osteoclasts. Regular exercise also helps contribute to the alkalinity of blood and tissue fluids. By increasing the excretion of acid waste through perspiration and by increasing carbon dioxide output through expiration, regular exercise can tilt the pH of tissue fluids toward alkalinity.

2. Wise use of supplements. Bone acts as a reserve of minerals for the body, and proper intake of minerals is important to maintain what our bones need.

   a. Calcium is essential for human life and the functioning of every cell in our body. The National Institutes of Health announced that most women in the United States are not getting enough calcium in their diets. Their recommendation was from 1,000 to 1,500 mg per day in order to stem osteoporosis.

   b. Vitamin D is one of the most important regulators of calcium. It enhances intestinal calcium absorption and decreases the excretion of calcium in the kidneys. One can get vitamin D either directly from the diet or a supplement. In general, 400 to 800 IU is considered effective. However, the body converts cholesterol into vitamin D in the skin when exposed to natural sunlight. Ten minutes of sun exposure a day (without sunscreen) meets typical needs for vitamin D.

   c. All human cells contain magnesium, totaling about 25,000 mg in the body of an adult. About 60 to 70 percent of the body's magnesium is stored in the bones. Magnesium is necessary for calcium utilization, and it protects against the accumulation of calcium deposits in the urinary tract. Such deposits may otherwise lead to bladder or kidney stones. Based on the percentages of magnesium in bones from patients with osteoporosis (0.62 percent) and healthy people (1.26 percent), magnesium plays an important role in bone hardness. The recommended dosage is 400 to 750 mg daily.

   d. Boron plays an important role in hardening bones. It is a new recruit in the battle against bone loss. This trace mineral has been found to reduce the excretion of calcium, magnesium, and phosphorus, thus retaining minerals necessary to keep bone hard. It also increases blood levels of active forms of estrogen and testosterone, which are important for maintaining healthy bones. Recommended dosage is 3 mg daily to help increase the absorption of calcium.

e. Add supplemental folic acid (400 to 800 mcg daily) and vitamin B-12 (500 to 1,000 mcg daily) for seniors with elevated levels of homocysteine, which has been linked to increased instances of hip fracture. Homocysteine does not affect bone density, but it can damage collagen, leading to weakened cross-linking between the collagen fibers that reinforce the bone tissue.

3. Change of lifestyle: Methods of preventing osteoporosis include a change of lifestyle. As discussed before, exercise and proper nutrition during adolescence are important for the prevention of osteoporosis. Exercise and nutrition throughout the rest of our lives delays bone degeneration. Individuals already diagnosed with osteopenia or osteoporosis should discuss their exercise program with their physician to avoid fractures. Some lifestyle choices increase the risk of osteoporosis, including:

a. Excess alcohol. Small amounts of alcohol do not increase osteoporosis risk, but chronic heavy drinking (alcohol intake greater than 3 units per day), especially at a younger age, increases the risks significantly.

b. Tobacco smoking. Tobacco smoking inhibits the activity of osteoblasts, thus reducing new bone formation. Smoking also results in increased breakdown of estrogen, which contributes to lower bone mineral density.

c.  Physical inactivity. Bone remodeling occurs in response to physical stress; thus, weight-bearing exercise can increase bone mass. Physical inactivity can lead to significant bone loss.

d.  Excess physical activity. Excessive exercise can damage the bones by causing stress to the bone structures. There are many examples of marathon runners who developed severe osteoporosis later in life. In women, intensive and strenuous exercise can lead to decreased estrogen levels, which predispose them to osteoporosis. Heavy training without proper compensatory nutrition raises the risk.

e.  Excess carbonated soft drinks. One average 8 oz can contains 136 mg of phosphorus, with no calcium. If you are "super sizing" your order, you consume 62 to 84 oz of soda, which may contain over 1,000 mg of phosphorus, with no calcium. If you have too much phosphorus in your blood, your body will pull calcium right out of your bones.

f.  Excess of highly processed foods. Increased dependency upon highly processed foods that are low in calcium and high in phosphorus has become more common in this busy world. The use of phosphate food additives (a binding agent that stops microbe growth) may cause calcium loss. Processed foods with labels containing ingredients like pyrophosphate, polyphosphate, sodium phosphate, and phosphoric acid significantly increase our dietary intake of phosphorus, without providing balancing calcium. Just like drinking too many carbonated soft drinks, overeating highly processed foods can also lead to net calcium loss. When a diet frequently contains a combination of soft drinks and TV dinners, the risk of osteoporosis is increased dramatically.

4. Certain medications are known to be associated with an increase in osteoporosis risk. Steroids, including prednisone; inhaled corticosteroids, like Advair or Flovent; and anticonvulsants, such as Dilantin, Klonopin, and Tegretol, are classically associated with osteoporosis, but evidence is emerging with regard to other drugs. High-dose thyroid hormones like Levoxyt or Synthroid may contribute to osteoporosis. Long-term use of anticoagulants, such as heparin, warfarin, and coumarins, has been linked with an increased risk in osteoporotic fractures. Prolonged use of proton pump inhibitors, such as Prevacid and Prilosec, which are used to inhibit the production of stomach acid, can interfere with calcium absorption, leading to increased risk of osteoporosis due to calcium deficiency. Concerns about long-term use of these medications should be seriously considered, especially if you have low bone density.

A recent study (*Obstetrics and Gynecology*, January 2010) that followed women who used the birth control method Depo-Provera every three months found that 45 percent of users experienced bone mineral density losses of 5 percent or more in the hip or lower spine within two years. More than two million women use Depo-Provera, including about 400,000 teenagers. Researchers concluded that the bone loss after Depo-Provera use was of significant concern, because it takes a long time for bone mass to recover, and the hip is the most common fracture site in women late in life.

As we can see, more than one risk factor is involved in the development of osteoporosis. There is a great deal we can do naturally and nutritionally to enhance bone health and to prevent osteoporotic fractures. Any one measure or one drug does not guarantee a total protective effect against osteoporotic fractures. By bringing your body back to optimal physiological condition at a healthy pH of 7.4 in tissue fluids, increasing the body's alkaline reserve, you can forestall losing calcium compounds from the bones. With the proper intake of essential minerals, you can maintain what the bone needs. By changing your lifestyle, modifying your nutritional profile, and avoiding certain medications known to cause osteoporosis, you can gradually reach a balance between bone resorption and bone formation. This whole-body approach combines all the anti-osteoporosis measures that deal with various risk factors. All these measures work together synergistically to protect your bone health and to increase your chance of success. It's never too late to improve your bone health and prevent osteoporotic fractures.

# Chapter 8
# Can Age-Related Cancer Be Prevented?

Cancer is a disease in which a group of cells grows uncontrollably, destroys adjacent tissue, and sooner or later spreads to other locations in the body via lymph or blood. These three properties distinguish cancers from benign tumors, which are self-limited and do not invade adjacent tissue or spread to other locations. With the exception of leukemia, most cancers form a tumor mass because cancer cells divide more frequently and live longer than normal cells, clumping and accumulating to form a mass. They compete with the surrounding healthy tissue for oxygen and nutrients in the blood, crowding out healthy cells and inhibiting normal physiological functions.

In the United States, cancer is responsible for 25 percent of all deaths; 30 percent of those are from lung cancer. The most commonly occurring cancer in men is prostate cancer; in women it is breast cancer. According to the American Cancer Society, the most common types of cancer in terms of the approximate number of new cases per year are: prostate, breast, lung, colon and rectum, lymphoma, bladder, and melanoma. The most frequent causes of cancer-related deaths are: lung, colon and rectum, breast, prostate, pancreas, and lymphoma. This discrepancy is simply due to different behaviors among different types of cancer. Some types of cancer are more aggressive and harder to treat than others and thus are more likely to be fatal. Lung cancer is by far the most deadly form of malignant tumor. Although prostate cancer is the most common type of cancer in terms of the number of cases, it is less often the cause of death than some other forms of cancer.

As of 2004, worldwide cancer caused 13 percent of all deaths for a total of 7.4 million (*Cancer*, World Health Organization). The leading causes of cancer-related deaths were lung, stomach, colon and rectum, liver, and breast. The variation of cancer-related deaths in the United States as compared to other parts of world is mainly due to the different risk factors present in different countries.

In the United States, one in four people will develop cancer during their lifetime; after heart disease, cancer is the second-leading cause of death. Each year more than 1.6 million Americans develop cancer. In fact, cancer is on the rise, mainly because the risks for most cancers increase with age, and Americans are living longer. A rapid increase in the number of lung cancer deaths has boosted the rate of cancer deaths, even though death rates from cancer of the uterus, stomach, and liver have declined significantly. In recent years there have been significant improvements in survival times. Today, more than 50 percent of people with cancer survive five years or longer, an improvement largely due to earlier detection and improved treatment.

**Some Unique Problems in Cancer Diagnosis**

Cancer has a reputation for being a deadly disease. This certainly applies to certain types of cancer, such as small cell carcinoma of the lung, and a cancer diagnosis has a substantial impact on a cancer patient's quality of life and an emotional impact on family members. However, some types of cancer have a prognosis that is substantially better than serious nonmalignant diseases, such as heart failure and stroke. Furthermore, particular types of cancer, such as carcinoid of the lung, can even be considered a low-grade malignancy that can be cured after initial treatment. It is therefore extremely important to obtain an accurate diagnosis.

Most cancers are initially recognized either by signs or symptoms or through screening. Neither of these leads to a definitive diagnosis. People with suspected cancer undergo further medical tests, commonly including blood tests, X-rays, CT scans, and endoscopy. After such examinations, a cancer may be suspected for a variety of reasons, but the definitive diagnosis of most malignant tumors must be confirmed by cytological and/or histological examination of the cancerous cells or tissues by a pathologist. Tissue can be obtained by fine-needle aspiration or surgical biopsy. If the lesion is not palpable, then the biopsy needs the guidance of an imaging technique, such as ultrasound or CT scan.

The tissue diagnosis provided by the pathologist indicates the type of malignant cells, the histological grade, genetic abnormalities, and other features of the tumor. Cytogenetics and immunohistochemistry are other types of testing that the pathologist may perform on the specimen. These tests may provide information about changes at the molecular level, such as mutations, fusion genes, and numerical chromosome changes that have occurred in the cancer cells, as well as indicate the future behavior of the cancer and the treatment of choice. All this information is useful for evaluating the prognosis of the cancer and choosing the best treatment.

Cancer is not something that just happens over a short period of time. It takes many years for normal epithelial cells to become dysplastic cells and to progress to cancer cells. The natural history of certain cancers, such as cervical cancer of the uterus, has been studied in great detail. Based on the findings of microscopic examinations, invasive squamous cell carcinomas of the uteri cervix are invariably preceded by this sequence: squamous metaplasia of endocervical epithelium, to dysplasia (mild, moderate, to severe degree of nuclear abnormalities), to carcinoma in situ (CIS, intraepithelial lesion only), to invasive squamous cell carcinoma. Dysplasia of a mild or moderate degree is considered a reversible process. Follow-up after conservative therapy has shown regression in 62 percent of cases, persistence in 22 percent, and progression to a severe lesion in 16 percent. Severe dysplasia and CIS are actively proliferating lesions that, if left alone, will eventually evolve to invasive cancer. They rarely regress, may persist for long periods, and are generally accepted as a precursor of invasive cervical cancer (Rosai, J., *Ackerman's Surgical Pathology.* Mosby, 1989). The average timing from squamous metaplasia to mild dysplasia, to moderate and then to severe dysplasia, to CIS, and ultimately to invasive cancer, takes twenty years.

When I was at the Toronto General Hospital in Toronto, Canada, during the nineteen seventies and eighties, I worked with thoracic surgeons on smoking-related lung cancer (squamous cell carcinoma). We observed that it took, on average, thirty-seven years for metaplastic squamous epithelial cells of the bronchus to become dysplastic cells (mild, moderate, to severe degree) and to progress to CIS cells and ultimately to cancer cells (*Cancer*, 50: 1580–86, 1982). The causative agents are different in cervical cancer and lung cancer. In uteri cervix, the cancer is induced by human papillomavirus and in the lung by tobacco smoke carcinogens. This may explain the different durations in the development of the same type of cancer.

In fact, 90 percent of human bodies carry precancerous dysplastic cells, which are induced by chemical carcinogens, ionizing radiation, viral infection, or free radical attacks. If the body's immune system is in optimal condition, immune cells can recognize these dysplastic cells as foreign invaders and get rid of them before they progress to cancer cells. Many authors on aging report that 90 percent of us carry cancer cells in our bodies. From a pathologist's point of view, this statement is incorrect and misleading and may cause unnecessary apprehension and alarm among the general public.

## Causative Factors in Developing Age-Related Cancers

Less than 10 percent of all cancer types are due to an inherited predisposition and are usually seen in younger age groups. Far more common, especially among seniors who have an increased risk of age-related cancer, are the carcinogenic mutations of somatic (body) cells, which crop up as a result of continual environmental insults, including chemical carcinogens and ionizing radiation. Substances that cause DNA mutations are known as mutagens, and mutagens that cause cancers are known as carcinogens. There are also naturally occurring carcinogens, such as toxins from some molds. Viral infections may also cause cancer. The following are causative factors commonly noted in age-related cancers:

1. Chemical carcinogens. Tobacco smoking is associated with many forms of cancer and causes 90 percent of lung cancer. Decades of research has demonstrated the direct or contributory link between tobacco use and cancer in the lung, larynx, stomach, bladder, kidney, esophagus, and pancreas. Tobacco smoke contains over fifty known carcinogens, including nitrosamines and polycyclic aromatic hydrocarbons. Prolonged exposure to asbestos fibers is associated with mesothelioma. Environmental pollutants pose a persistent risk. The link between cancer and exposure to industrial dyes, nickel, chromate, vinyl chloride, toxins from some molds, and benzene has been well established.

2. Ionizing radiation. Sources of ionizing radiation, such as radon gas, can cause cancer. Prolonged exposure to ultraviolet radiation from the sun can lead to malignant melanoma and other skin malignant tumors. A report published in *Lancet Oncology* (August, 2009) found that when the use of tanning

devices starts before age thirty, the risk of melanoma increases 75 percent. It also found consistent evidence of a link between melanoma of the eye and the use of tanning devices. Ionized particles are highly active and can damage other molecules, including molecules of DNA. The cancer risk due to current CT scans, which contain ionizing radiation at levels much higher than that of diagnostic X-rays, is still uncertain. During a chest X-ray, the patient is exposed to 20 to 40 mrem of radiation. A chest CT using an electron beam CT scanner involves 125 to 160 mrem (scans of the abdomen plus pelvis add 160 to 200 mrem). A chest CT using a helical CT scanner involves 500 to 700 mrem (scans of the abdomen plus pelvis add 800 to 1,000 mrem). However, for occupational exposure, the safe limit is 5,000 mrem per year.

3. Viral infection. Many cancers originate from a viral infection. The viruses associated with human cancers include human immunodeficiency virus (HIV, causing acquired immunodeficiency syndrome: AIDS, which is associated with Kaposi's sarcoma), human papillomavirus (cervical cancer of the uterus, cancer of the base of the tongue, and cancer of the tonsils), hepatitis B and hepatitis C virus (liver cancer), and Epstein-Barr virus (nasopharyngeal carcinoma). Herpes simplex virus (HSV-2), which causes genital herpes, may be a cofactor in the risk for cervical cancer.

4. Free radical attacks. This recently recognized causative factor in developing cancer was rarely discussed in the past. In fact, this risk factor is especially important for seniors, because the production of endogenous superoxide dismutase (a powerful free radical killer) greatly decreases with age. As discussed before, when mitochondria in cells convert nutrients into energy, they generate numerous corrosive free radicals at the same time. There are hundreds of mitochondria per cell. Free radicals are

also produced as part of many other enzymatic reactions that our body performs to sustain life. In addition, free radicals are created in very high levels throughout the body whenever there is trauma, infection, or inflammation. Chronic cigarette smoking and chronic alcohol drinking also produce high levels of free radicals. Free radicals, which act like highly reactive oxygen molecules, may react with nucleic acid. Every cell in our body receives an estimated 10,000 free radical hits daily. Those intracellular free radical attacks can cause cell deaths or mutations that incite cells to aberrant behavior, resulting in precancerous dysplastic cells. In fact, 90 percent of us, especially seniors, carry dysplastic cells in various organs. In people with a weakened immune system, these dysplastic cells can progress to cancer cells. Free radical attacks could be the most important causative factor in developing cancer among seniors, because profuse intracellular free radicals are continuously created.

5.  Immune system dysfunction. HIV is associated with a number of malignant tumors, including Kaposi's sarcoma and lymphoma. The increased incidence of malignant tumors in HIV patients points to the breakdown of immune system as a possible etiology of cancer. Certain other immune deficiency conditions, such as IgA deficiency and undergoing immunosuppressive therapy, are also associated with increased cancer risk. Chronic stress, whether it stems from external pressure or internal perception, also impairs immunity. Alcoholics and people who experience higher levels of stress have suppressed immune systems and tend to have an increased risk of developing cancer.

## The Whole-Body Approach to Reducing Risks of Age-Related Cancer

As mentioned above, only a small portion of all cancer types—perhaps less than 10 percent—are due to an inherited predisposition. However, having a predisposition does not necessarily mean that a person will develop cancer. The vast majority of age-related cancers are due to carcinogenic mutations of certain types of body cells that occur within the individual's life and arise as a result of environmental or lifestyle-related risk factors or endogenous, intracellular free radical attacks.

Nonetheless, some pharmaceutical companies would like you to believe that the genetic factor plays an important role in the development of cancer and is not preventable by any natural or nutritional means. They, perhaps, want you to think your only hope is to give up and just trust their latest drugs. One such drug, Avastin, once received a lot of attention in the media and among the public. It is the world's best-selling cancer drug, with global sales of $5.8 billion, and it costs about $8,000 a month. After three years of medical use, federal regulators recently took the step of moving to revoke approval of Avastin to treat advanced breast cancer. According to Janet Woodcock, director of the FDA's Center for Drug Evaluation and Research, after careful review of the clinical data from four independent studies, new evidence clearly demonstrated that patients receiving Avastin did not live longer and also experienced a significant increase in serious side effects, including blood clots, bleeding, and heart failure.

More and more evidence suggests that age-related cancers are largely preventable. A major study, the European Prospective Investigation into Cancer and Nutrition, which monitored more than 470,000 people in ten different countries, found that the risk for colon cancer was twice as high for people who ate large quantities of red meat (a strongly acidifying food) as for those who consumed fewer than 20 g a day (*Journal of the National Cancer Institute*, No.12, 2005). In another study by the Department of Epidemiology at Harvard University that followed 91,000 nurses over twelve years, researchers reached the same conclusion for breast cancer. They found that the risk of breast cancer in women was twice as high in those who ate red meat more than once a day as for those who consumed it less than three times a week (Servan-Schreiber, D., *Anticancer*. Viking, 2008).

Proposed dietary interventions for cancer risk reduction gain support from epidemiological studies (Beliveau, R. and Gingras, D., *Foods That Fight Cancers*. McClelland and Stewart, 2006). Such studies include reports that reduced red meat consumption is associated with decreased risk of colon cancer. A cancer prevention study found that consumption of a plant-based diet plus lifestyle changes resulted in a reduction in cancer markers (PSA) in a group of men with prostate cancer who were using no conventional treatments at the time. Recent studies have also demonstrated potential links between some forms of cancer (including breast, kidney, pancreas, and prostate cancers) and high consumption of refined sugars and refined grains, both of which are also acidifying foods.

All these studies appear to indicate that heavy and prolonged consumption of red meat, refined sugar, and/or refined grains, all of which are acidifying foods, increases the acidity in the tissue fluids (even though the pH of the blood remains 7.4), resulting in the development of cancer. Following a long period of acidic tissue fluids, various physiological functions of the body, including immune function, deteriorate, allowing precancerous dysplastic cells to progress to cancer cells and then to proliferate.

There is a great deal you can do through natural means and nutrition to restore the acid-alkaline balance in the tissue fluids, to boost the immune system, and to control free radical attacks, thereby reducing the production of precancerous dysplastic cells and curtailing their progression to cancer cells. The whole-body approach is intended to allow the whole body to work synergistically to prevent the development of age-related cancer.

1. Bring your body back to optimal physiological condition, with a healthy pH of 7.4 in tissue fluids to increase the body's alkaline reserve. Your body can then use the alkaline reserve to neutralize the acid products from the digestion of meat and other acidifying foods, stabilizing the acid-alkaline balance in the tissue fluids. The self-healing power of the human body is effective only if the body is in optimal physiological condition. By restoring the acid-alkaline balance of tissue fluids to a healthy pH of 7.4, the human body's physiological functions can perform at the optimal level, including isolating and killing precancerous dysplastic cells.

Suggested measures

a. Have a glass of freshly squeezed vegetable and fruit juice (200 to 250 ml) every morning. Choose five or six from the following list: celery, onion, cucumber, zucchini, carrot, radish, green apple, green papaya, and pear. The amount of each variety can be adjusted to your taste. Make your own recipe. This measure boosts alkaline reserves.

b. If your morning fasting saliva pH test indicates an acidic pH, eat 20 percent acidifying foods and 80 percent alkalizing foods every day until the pH of your morning fasting saliva pH test ranges between 7.2 and 7.6. You may then increase acidifying foods to 30 percent if you wish. You can make use of the pH reading of morning fasting saliva pH test as a guide to adjust the various portions of acidifying and alkalizing foods.

c. Make sure that the water you drink from the same source every day has a pH close to 7.4 and contains minerals your body needs. Forget about carbonated soft drinks, especially those containing phosphates and large amounts of sugar, which are strongly acidifying and harmful.

d. Changes in lifestyle may help reduce the risk of age-related cancer. Large amounts of alcohol are acidifying, and chronic alcohol abuse can suppress the immune function. Alcohol impedes the ability of immune cells to identify precancerous dysplastic cells, which will readily multiply and develop into cancer. High alcohol consumption can increase the risk of oral, esophageal, and breast cancers. Physical inactivity is associated with increased risk of colon and breast cancers and obesity with colon, breast, and endometrial cancers. Other lifestyles known to affect cancer risk include certain sexually transmitted diseases, such as human papillomavirus infection, leading to uteri cervical cancer, cancer of tonsils, and cancer of the base of tongue.

2. Boost your immune system. A healthy immune system, well-armed with natural killer (NK) cells, T and B lymphocytes, leukocytes, plasma cells, and macrophages, is able to identify precancerous dysplastic cells and can eliminate them before they progress to cancer cells.

Suggested measures

a. Proper diet with necessary supplements. In order to enable the immune system to function optimally, the body needs to have sufficient amounts of vitamins A, B, C, D, E, and K (thirteen kinds altogether); various essential minerals and trace elements (sixteen kinds); eight essential amino acids; and two essential fatty acids. If for any reason you cannot eat a balanced and healthful diet, make up for the lack with a multivitamin pill and other supplements, such as omega-3 fish oil soft gels (1,000 to 2,000 mg) daily.

The National Cancer Institute and the American Cancer Society have agreed on dietary guidelines to help lower the risk of certain types of cancer. These recommendations include the following:

- Eat a well-balanced diet, including at least five portions of fresh fruits and vegetables (each portion should generally be one half cup or more) every day. Do not overcook vegetables because it diminishes their nutritional value. Steaming vegetables is the healthiest way of cooking, as it retains the most vitamins and minerals.

- Concentrate on foods in your diet that are high in vitamins A and C, including squash, carrots, sweet potatoes, spinach, apricots, and peaches. Foods that are high in vitamin C include oranges, strawberries, grapefruits, green peppers, red peppers, and broccoli. Studies have shown that vitamin A may lower the risk of certain cancers, including cancer of the larynx, pharynx, and lung. Vitamin C may act as an antioxidant and reduce the production of some carcinogenic compounds.

- Eat foods that are high in fiber. These include grains, whole grain breads, lentils, and legumes.

- Eat cruciferous vegetables, such as broccoli, cabbage, cauliflower, kale, Brussels sprouts, and Swiss chard. Some research shows that cruciferous vegetables may lower the risk of colon, stomach, and lung cancers.

- Cut down on the amount of saturated and polyunsaturated (omega-6) fat in your diet.

- Cut back on the amount of processed foods and foods containing nitrites.

- Cut back on the amount of smoked and salt-cured foods.

- Limit the amount of alcohol you consume to no more than two drinks a day.

b. Relieve stress. Chronic mental stress, whether it stems from external pressure or internal perception, also impairs immunity. Alcoholics and people who experience higher levels of stress tend to have suppressed immune system and are in danger of developing cancer. Stress-reduction measures, such as aerobic exercise, yoga, and tai chi, and other forms of relaxation, such as a hobby, massage, listening to music, and meditation, can be tried as a first step toward gaining control. Individual stress management consultations or programs are offered by some hospitals and medical schools.

c. Avoid environmental cancer risk factors, such as chemical carcinogens (including tobacco smoke, asbestos fibers, industrial dyes, nickel, chromate, vinyl chloride, formaldehyde, benzene, Bisphenol A, toxins from some molds, pesticides, and benzopyrene, heterocyclic amines from high-temperature cooking); ionizing radiation (including radon gas, and CT scans); and viral infections (including human immunodeficiency virus, human papillomavirus, hepatitis B and hepatitis C virus, and Epstein-Barr virus). At no other time in history has the human body been bombarded by so many adverse factors on a consistent basis. Yet cancer is not something that just happens over a short period of time. It takes many years for normal epithelial cells to progress to dysplastic cells and then to cancer cells. Fortunately, we do have plenty of time to safeguard our bodies against various carcinogenic attacks and to stop the progression of dysplastic cells to cancer cells.

3.  Control free radical attacks. This is especially important for seniors, because the production of endogenous superoxide dismutase, a powerful free radical killer, is greatly reduced as age advances. However, an abundance of free radicals are produced continuously as byproducts of many enzymatic reactions our body performs to sustain life. These intracellular free radicals can attack DNA and cause cell mutations that incite cells to aberrant behavior, emerging as precancerous dysplastic cells. Thus the burden is on us to safeguard our bodies from free radical attacks and curtail the progression of dysplastic cells to cancer cells. Antioxidants for this purpose are preferably those which can be transported across cell membranes into mitochondria, where intracellular free radicals are commonly produced. Wise use of antioxidants can help control free radical attacks.

    a.  Alpha lipoic acid. It is the only fat- and water-soluble antioxidant, easily absorbed and transported across cell membranes, eliminating free radicals both inside and outside cells. It has the ability to enhance the antioxidant power of vitamins C, E, and glutathione in the body, creating an antioxidant network that provides more protection against damaging free radicals. The recommended dosage is 100 to 200 mg daily.

    b.  Coenzyme Q10 (CoQ10). This substance can actually penetrate into the mitochondria and is an essential component of the metabolic process involved in energy production. It can stimulate immunity. Unfortunately, the body's production of CoQ10 begins to decline around age twenty and is seriously deficient by middle age. The recommended dosage for seniors is 100 to 300 mg daily. CoQ10 has virtually no side effects at any dose.

c.  Melatonin. This hormone is made from the amino acid tryptophan. The body converts the tryptophan into the neurotransmitter serotonin, and then at night serotonin is converted into melatonin in the pineal gland. Melatonin ranks as one of the important hormones, and it is also a powerful antioxidant. However, levels of melatonin greatly decrease as we age. Melatonin can boost the immune system by strengthening antibody response and increasing immune cell activity. It increases the immune system's ability to spot and destroy precancerous dysplastic cells. The recommended dosage is 1 to 5 mg daily, depending on age. It is important that melatonin only be taken at night, about a half to one hour before bed. Although melatonin is harmless to the body and causes no side effects, it is not recommended for people under forty years of age, to avoid prematurely interfering with your own production of the hormone.

d.  Quercetin. This is a natural free radical killer found in onion and garlic. It can slow the development of cancer through its protective action against the damage caused by carcinogenic substances and its ability to prevent cancer cell growth. But quercetin is very soluble in water, and it can be easily eliminated by rinsing peeled bulbs under running water and by cooking. It is better to soak an onion in red wine, to fully preserve quercetin. This way, onion and red wine work together synergistically to further enhance the valuable anticancer effects.

There is a great deal we can do naturally and nutritionally to reduce the risk of age-related cancer. Firstly, by strictly controlling intracellular free radical attacks, the production of precancerous dysplastic cells is greatly reduced or avoided. Secondly, by boosting your immune system to optimal condition, the immune cells can recognize these dysplastic cells as foreign invaders and get rid of them before they progress to cancer cells. Thirdly, by bringing up the pH of tissue fluids to a healthy level of 7.4, which indicates an optimal physiological condition, you create an environment inhospitable to the growth of cancer cells. The whole-body approach is intended to let the entire body work together synergistically to protect your health and to reduce the risk of age-related cancer. Any one measure or a few supplements do not guarantee protection against cancer.

# Chapter 9
# Protecting Your Brain and Keeping It Healthy

The brain is our body's most complex organ and one of the busiest and most metabolically active organs in the body. It is composed of a compact network of more than ten billion nerve cells. It weighs less than three pounds and represents less than 2 percent of total body weight; yet it contains 15 percent of the body's total blood flow, uses 25 percent of its oxygen, and consumes 70 percent of its glucose.

The health of the brain and body are closely related and go hand in hand. One cannot proceed without the other. Just like other organs, the brain needs nutrients, fuel, and even exercise to keep it functioning properly, thereby enhancing thinking, elevating mood, and boosting memory. However, it also has unique aspects and is different from other organs in the following respects:

1.  The brain is not capable of storing its own supply of nutrients and energy. It relies on a constant flow of blood to keep it nutritionally replenished. It must have a continual supply of glucose, oxygen, and other essential nutrients.

2. The brain must depend on glucose from the blood for energy and most of its metabolic activities, while other organs in the body can metabolize glycogen, fat, and even protein for energy supply.

3. Without the proper supply of special nutrients directly to the brain, some neurotransmitters, which are special brain chemicals, required by nerve cells to maintain proper brain function cannot be produced, leading to impairment of mental functions such as memory, mood, and thinking.

4. The brain has a special apparatus to pump glucose from the blood into the brain across a unique blood-brain barrier. This barrier prevents most large molecules and toxic substances in the blood from entering brain tissue, keeping many potentially damaging substances out of the brain. This protective mechanism may also keep some large-molecule nutrients and medicines from entering.

5. The brain, which consists of 60 percent fats (though it cannot store fat as an energy supply) and elevated levels of polyunsaturated fats (omega-3 and omega-6 fatty acids), the target of lipid peroxidation, also has a high metabolic rate and is uniquely vulnerable to oxidative injuries from increased free radical attacks and oxidative stress.

Because of this unique brain physiology, biochemistry, and pathology, therapeutic intervention for many chronic neurodegenerative diseases is more difficult and generally less effective. It has become clear that age-related changes in the brain are greatly influenced by the biochemical environment of the brain. Many nutrients and natural substances can have a favorable impact on that biochemical environment in relation to brain function. The brain is greatly influenced by what you eat. The quality of the nutrients and supplements fed to the brain directly impacts a person's ability to think and remember, as well as the person's mood.

Age-related decline in brain function, such as memory impairment, senile dementia, mental deterioration, and cognitive decline among seniors, is extremely common and sometimes becomes a serious health problem. Furthermore, many seniors are taking a wide variety of prescription and over-the-counter medications that may adversely affect mental function and cause mood swings, even depression. Brain cells are generally more sensitive than other body cells to nutrients and dietary chemicals that may determine how your brain functions or malfunctions. It is therefore extremely important to protect your brain from nutritional deficiencies and keep it healthy in order to maintain quality of life in your senior years.

By the year 2030, eighty million Americans will be older than sixty-five. The aging of the population is spurring a new realization that a vital body without a vital brain is meaningless (Carper, J., *Your Miracle Brain*. Harper, 2000). We must start paying as much, or even more, attention to the brain as we do to the heart. It is never too late to improve the health of your brain, boosting its functioning to the optimal intellectual and emotional heights.

With the inventions of sophisticated brain imaging, including positron-emission tomography (PET), magnetic resonance imaging (MRI), and single photon emission-computed tomography (SPECT), we can track the workings of a living human brain. This has ushered in a new era of understanding the real "biology of the brain." New research has proven that adult brains, contrary to previous beliefs, can grow new nerve cells that are able to produce new dendrites and receptors and grow new synapses, the communication junctions between nerve cells. For the first time in human history, scientists are beginning to understand how profoundly food, supplements, and lifestyle changes can influence brain function. New research also shows that nutrients, including glucose and fat, can have an almost immediate impact on brain cells and brain functioning, producing rapid changes in mood and long-term behavior.

## Understanding Neurons and Neurotransmitters

At the core of our intellect, our memory, and our emotions are nerve cells called neurons. A neuron is a cell with roundish body, a large nucleus, and offshoots of a complex bushy network of dendrites—sinewy branches studded with countless surface receptors—and a single long nerve fiber called an axon. The receptors on the dendrites receive incoming signals from other neurons, which streak down the dendritic branches to the cell body where the information is processed and are then passed on to the axon for transmission to other neurons through synaptic connections. At the end of the axon is the storage terminal with tiny sacs full of neurotransmitters. As neurotransmitters are released, messages flash across synapses at the end of the axon of one cell to specific receptors on another. These receptors are shaped to receive only one type of neurotransmitter, which fits them like a key in a lock. These synapses are the message transmission centers of the neurons.

Each neuron can have myriad synapses and thus communicate with hundreds of thousands of other neurons in microseconds. The more strong synapses and dendrites a nerve cell has, the greater its capacity for transmitting messages and processing information. That transmission allows us to think, feel, remember, and dream. In healthy young people, the number of synaptic connections in the brain has been roughly estimated at a hundred billion. When dendrites thin out, neuronal transmission becomes inefficient or even comes to a halt. In addition, neurotransmitters may be in short supply due to lack of raw materials, or they may be blocked from reaching their proper receptors as a result of either genetics or certain chemicals. The malfunction of neurotransmitters then results in neurological problems.

With age, the number of dendrites and the synaptic density in certain regions of the brain, like the hippocampus, which is important for thinking, decrease. As a result, the brain's signal transmission slows down. This may explain almost all the age-related changes in cognitive abilities. Although there is some loss of synaptic connectivity in an aged brain, there is not much nerve-cell loss.

Neurotransmitters are special brain chemicals that form the biochemical electrification system of the brain. It is these brain chemicals that define who you are at every second of your life. Neurotransmitters flash through neurons one after another one in one direction, carrying your every thought and feeling through the brain's vast neuronal network. These neurotransmitters are either excitatory or inhibitory. If an excitatory neurotransmitter reaches the specific receptor, the nerve cell tends to fire. On the contrary, if an inhibitory neurotransmitter reaches the specific receptor, the nerve cell does not fire.

Communication within the brain, as well as between the brain and the rest of the nervous system, occurs through many different neurotransmitters and electrical impulses. The transmission of these impulses from one neuron to the others is achieved both chemically and electrically. Different parts of the brain contain different concentrations of various neurotransmitters. When these balances are disrupted, a variety of neurologic and psychiatric diseases may occur. Here are some major and extensively studied neurotransmitters of the brain:

1. **Serotonin** is the most extensively studied neurotransmitter. It affects practically every aspect of brain activities, helping shape your mood and outlook on life, as well as enhancing your memory and energy level. Low levels of serotonin have been implicated in depression, obsessive-compulsive disorder, schizophrenia, extreme violence, autism, social phobias, premenstrual syndrome, migraines, anxiety, and panic attacks. Serotonin's inhibitory effect in the brain prevents excess nervous stimulation at night; thus, sleep can more easily occur. Research

found that women synthesize serotonin at half the rate of men. This finding may help explain why women are more prone to depression. Serotonin circuits also become weaker with age simply because neurons lose the dendritic receptors needed to activate serotonin. The brains of sixty-five-year-olds have 60 percent fewer serotonin receptors than those of thirty-year-olds. The effect of serotonin decreases with age, thus increasing the tendency to depression. Therefore, increasing your serotonin levels can be important for emotional health.

Serotonin is synthesized directly from the essential amino acid tryptophan, with the assistance of vitamin B-6 and carbohydrates. Researchers at the Massachusetts Institute of Technology discovered that the serotonin concentration in the brain is directly proportional to the concentration of plasma tryptophan. This demonstrates the feasibility of direct dietary control of a brain neurotransmitter, serotonin, by supplementation with tryptophan, a single essential amino acid.

2. **Dopamine** plays an important role in the control of movement. It has a stimulating effect on the heart and the metabolic rate and is able to mobilize many of the body's energy reserves. It helps modulate brain activity, control coordination of movement, and regulate the flow of information to different areas of the brain. It is widespread in the brain, as well as the rest of the nervous system. Dopamine is believed to induce the release of specific chemicals (e.g. endorphins), allowing us to feel pleasure, attachment, and love and to integrate thoughts. A severe disturbance of dopamine regulation in the brain can result in a person not being able to respond emotionally or express his or her feelings in an appropriate way, as in patients with schizophrenia. Abnormalities in dopamine concentration in parts of the brain lead to Parkinson's disease.

The main precursor for dopamine is the amino acid tyrosine; other nutrients, including folic acid, niacin, iron, and vitamin B-6, are necessary cofactors. Although tyrosine is a nonessential amino acid that our body is able to create, deficiencies in the production of tyrosine can occur. In such cases, increasing dietary supplementation may be necessary.

3. **Acetylcholine** was the first neurotransmitter ever defined. It is found in both the central nervous system and the peripheral nervous system. It is the primary neurotransmitter involved in thought, learning, and memory. It sharpens our concentration and perception. Acetylcholine also plays an important role in sending messages from motor neurons to muscles, especially the heart, bladder, and stomach. Myasthenia gravis, a disease characterized by generalized muscular weakness and fatigue, is caused by a faulty immune response against acetylcholine receptors.

   To manufacture acetylcholine, our bodies need choline, which is a component of lecithin (phosphatidyl choline), the richest source of choline and popularly known as a "nerve food." A lack of acetylcholine can produce a decline in memory. Foods that contain choline include liver, egg yolk, cheese, nuts, oatmeal, and soybeans. Drugs and medications can interfere with the manufacture and effectiveness of acetylcholine. Patients with Alzheimer's disease, which is characterized by severe disturbance in brain function, show a marked shortage of acetylcholine.

4. **Gamma-aminobutyric acid (GABA)** is an inhibitory neurotransmitter in the central nervous system that plays a role in regulating neuronal excitability throughout the nervous system. It helps the neurons recover after transmission, reducing anxiety and stress. It is a significant mood modulator. GABA is synthesized from glutamate in different parts of the body, but glutamate is poorly carried across the protective blood-brain

barrier. However, L-glutamine ("L" refers to a natural form of the glutamine) can cross the blood-brain barrier more readily; once it crosses the barrier, it is quickly converted to glutamate. Supplementation with L-glutamine not only increases the level of GABA in the brain, it also serves as "fuel" for the brain.

Neurotransmitters play an important role in brain functions, and their proper levels in the brain are essential to maintaining a good quality of life. Low neurotransmitter levels produced in the neurons cause the postsynaptic neurons to fire ineffectively or not at all. Neurotransmitters are fat-soluble and cannot penetrate the blood-brain barrier. They can only be synthesized on site in the neurons with raw materials that are able to cross the barrier. GABA is an example. Supplementation with L-glutamine rather than glutamate, which is a precursor of GABA but penetrates the blood-brain barrier poorly, increases the level of GABA in the brain.

## Primary Causes of Age-Related Loss of Cognitive Ability

The brain is subject to the same basic biology as the rest of the body: from built-in senescence to normal wear and tear to damage by free radicals. As a result, the brain undergoes dramatic changes as the decades pile up. The average fifty-year-old's brain weighs three pounds; fifteen years later it weighs 2.6 lbs. Gaps between the folds of cortex and the large spaces inside the brain enlarge, followed by loss of cognitive ability. The primary causes of loss of cognitive ability in seniors follow:

1. Most of brain shrinkage comes from lost intracellular tissue fluid. The frontal lobes, the site of higher thought, including problem solving, abstract thinking, and multitasking, show more thinning than any other part of the brain. On average, they shrink 30 percent between the ages of fifty and ninety. Nutritional deficiencies also contribute to the brain shrinkage process. The hippocampus, a small sea-horse-shaped structure

in the rear part of the brain, crucial to forming and retrieving memories, can lose about 20 percent of its volume between the ages fifty and ninety, resulting in cognitive ability losses.

2.  The myelin sheath that insulates the axons of the neurons is made of polyunsaturated fatty acids (omega-3 and omega-6 fatty acids), the target of lipid peroxidation, and is vulnerable to oxidative injuries from free radical attacks and oxidative stress. Brain tissue has a high rate of metabolism, and that also generates more free radicals. The higher level of free radical attacks increases the degradation of myelin sheath, which reduces the velocity at which electrical signals zip around the brain. The reduced conduction velocity of axons, which slows down information processing, occurs frequently in aging brains.

3.  Although brain shrinkage mostly reflects loss of intracellular tissue fluid, it is also the result of shrinking dendrites and reduced synapses, due to increased free radical attacks in the aging brain. When dendrites and synapses are numerous and strong, there is greater neuron-to-neuron transmission. It is this transmission that lets us think, feel, and remember. With age, the numbers of dendrites and synapses in a given area decrease, leaving the brain less connected. When dendrites and synapses thin out, neuronal transmission is reduced or even halted, followed by loss of cognitive ability.

4.  In seniors with high blood pressure, diabetes, and heart disease, fatty deposits and scar tissue slowly accumulate in the linings of blood vessels, reducing blood flow to various organs, including the brain, usually due to narrowing of the carotid arteries. Decreased blood flow to the brain reduces nutrients and the oxygen supply that the brain needs for maintaining a high rate of metabolism and manufacturing neurotransmitters. This can

eventually lead to lower levels of neurotransmitter production in the brain, slowing down neuronal signal transmission.

5.  Suppression of the central nervous system due to stress, worries, and/or pressure impairs brain functions. Mental stress can trigger the production of the stress hormone cortisol. High levels of cortisol can influence many aspects of brain activity. Chronic stress can reduce axon spouting and dendrite branching, both of which underlie learning and memory.

6.  Improper lifestyle, such as smoking, abusing alcohol, or using illegal drugs, can also affect brain health. Cigarette smoking impairs pulmonary and cardiac function, thus reducing oxygen and blood supply to the brain. Heavy alcohol consumption can cause the death of brain neurons. Illegal drugs can gradually deplete some of the neurotransmitters, or block them from reaching their proper receptors.

### The Whole-Body Approach to Reduce Risks of Age-Related Loss of Cognitive Ability

We have considerable control of our lives during our senior years. For most of us, long-term quality of life is driven neither by fate nor genetic disposition but by the choices we make today. It's now clear that senility is not inevitable. By providing sufficient special nutrients that the brain needs, controlling free radical attacks, and making lifestyle changes, you can keep your brain functioning properly and reduce the risk of age-related loss of cognitive ability. Here's how to gain an edge in protecting your brain and keeping it healthy.

1.  **Provide Sufficient Special and Essential Nutrients for Optimal Brain Function.** What is good for the heart also tends to be good for the brain, because unobstructed vessels will also supply sufficient oxygen and nutrients to your brain. The health of your brain and body go hand in hand. One cannot proceed without the other. With a healthy cardiovascular

system and proper supplementation of special nutrients for the brain, you are on the right track for reducing the risks of mental deterioration and cognitive decline. In the first place, you need to reduce the risk of cardiovascular disease, as discussed in chapter 6, and receive treatment for any hypertension, diabetes, and cardiovascular disease so as to improve your cardiovascular health. In addition to essential nutrients your body needs for optimal immune function, as discussed in chapter 3, your brain also needs some special nutrients in order to function optimally. The following are some of the ways to enhance thinking, elevate mood, and boost memory.

**A. Essential nutrients for optimal brain function.** Scientific evidence has linked nutrition and cognition. Numerous studies have confirmed that some vitamin deficiencies can cause mental problems at any age, and those with senility are more likely to have nutritional deficiencies. Researchers are now focusing on what is called *subclinical malnutrition*, a relatively mild nutritional deficiency. This nutritional deficiency generally manifests with very subtle symptoms, often related to brain functions such as intelligence and memory. Among all of the vitamins, the B vitamins and vitamin E are recognized to be essential for all aspects of the nervous system, including brain function. The B vitamins need to be taken together in adequate amounts throughout one's life.

*Thiamin (B-1): In the brain, it helps convert glucose into energy and plays a role in brain functions, including memory and cognition. The brain and nerves are the first areas of the body to show signs of vitamin B-1 deficiency. Symptoms include mental confusion, poor memory, difficulty in concentration, and even mental illness.

Recommended daily amount is 50 mg for men and 20 mg for women.

***Riboflavin (B-2):*** It helps with mental and cognitive ability in the brain. This is the most common vitamin deficiency of the brain. Symptoms of vitamin B-2 deficiency include trembling, lack of stamina and vigor, retarded growth, digestive problems, and even personality disturbances. Recommended daily amount is 50 mg for men and 20 mg for women.

***Niacin (B-3):*** In the brain, it enhances memory. As a person ages, the importance of this vitamin increases because it is very effective in restoring memory and improving energy levels and is useful in preventing or treating senility. Recommended daily amount is 100 mg for both men and women.

***Pantothenic Acid (B-5):*** It is essential to support the adrenal glands when a person is in stress and helps produce the antibodies that are needed to fight off infection. Symptoms of vitamin B-5 deficiency may include adrenal insufficiency, mental depression, excessive fatigue, nerve degenerative changes, palpitation, and gout. Recommended daily amount is 200 mg for both men and women.

***Pyridoxine (B-6):*** It is necessary for the manufacture of neurotransmitters. Symptoms of deficiency include numbness and tingling in hands and feet, neuritis, arthritis, low blood sugar, edema, mental retardation, excessive fatigue, nervous breakdown, mental illness, and epilepsy. In seniors, trembling in the hands is often noticed. Recommended daily amount is 50 mg for men and 30 mg for women.

**\*Cobalamin (B-12):** It plays an important role in the formation of the myelin sheath wrapping around nerve fibers. It is a common vitamin deficiency. Up to 50 percent of people age sixty and older experience seriously diminished hydrochloric acid (HCl) deficiency. A deficiency of HCl production in the stomach is known to impair vitamin B-12 and folic acid absorption. This may explain why vitamin B-12 and folic acid deficiencies are seen more often in seniors. Symptoms of vitamin B-12 deficiency include pernicious anemia; nerve dysfunction, such as muscle weakness, poor reflexes, and strange sensations in the arms and legs; and an impaired mental state. Many seniors have symptoms of intellectual impairment, manifested as difficulty in concentrating, poor memory for recent events, and difficulty at work. Some may have unsteadiness, excessive fatigue, a burning sensation, and even urinary incontinence. Recommended daily amount is 200 to 500 mcg for both men and women.

**\*Folic Acid:** It is necessary for the synthesis of DNA and RNA, which are required for new cell production. It is also a common vitamin deficiency in seniors, especially in patients with mental illness, including schizophrenia, dementia, and senility. Several researchers have reported that patients with symptoms of senility or dementia and low folic acid blood levels showed improvement after treatment with folic acid. A deficiency of folic acid during pregnancy has been linked to birth defects, one of the worst results of folic acid deficiency. Recommended daily amount is 400 mcg for both men and women.

**\*Tocopherol (vitamin E):** The brain is mostly fat (60 percent), making it extremely susceptible to fat-spoiling peroxidation. There is only one antioxidant, vitamin E, that dwells exclusively in the fatty part of cell membrane structures. Without sufficient vitamin E, the fatty parts of your brain, including mitochondria and outer cell membranes, are more apt to turn rancid, causing disturbances in the normal functioning of the neuron. Indeed, the first sign of a vitamin E deficiency is a neurological problem. Vitamin E helps regulate message transmission within cells as well as between cells. It is critical in directing and controlling activities of neurotransmitters once they enter the nerve cells. It also has immune-related benefits that reduce cell-damaging inflammation in the brain. Vitamin E fights plaque buildup and reduces clogging of blood vessels, improving oxygen and nutrient supply to the brain. Taking vitamin E helps prevent your carotid arteries from becoming blocked. Recommended daily amount of natural vitamin E is 400 to 500 IUs, considered adequate for good antioxidant protection.

**B. Special nutrients for the manufacture of major neurotransmitters in the brain.** Neurotransmitters are made up of amino acids. The type of neurotransmitters your neurons make and release within the brain is affected greatly by what you eat. Your brain cells need certain special nutrients as building blocks to make various neurotransmitters. The availability of a special nutrient in the brain can dictate the level of a particular neurotransmitter. The human brain is very capable of manufacturing needed quantities of neurotransmitters if it is given the raw materials to do so. However, a normal diet does not supply enough of the raw materials the brain needs to manufacture the optimal levels of some neurotransmitters. Additionally, stress, chemical use, poor nutrition, pollution, and other facts of modern life are known to deplete neurotransmitter levels. Thus, adding some special supplements for the brain in addition to a proper diet and essential B and E vitamin supplements seems necessary for good brain health. To make up for the lack, take some amino acid supplements, such as L-tryptophan, L-tyrosine, L-glutamine, and lecithin (phosphatidyl choline), every day.

* **L-tryptophan:** L-tryptophan acts as building blocks to make serotonin in the brain. Suggested daily amount is 500 mg. A modified form of tryptophan now available is called 5-HTP (5-hydroxytryptophan). 5-HTP is the direct precursor for making serotonin in the brain. Recommended daily amount is 200 to 300 mg.

***L-tyrosine:** L-tyrosine is a precursor for another important neurotransmitter, dopamine, and is found in foods containing high levels of protein. Very little tyrosine is found in cereals, vegetables, fruit, or oils. Recommended daily amount is 500 mg.

***L-glutamine:** As discussed before, L-glutamine can readily cross the blood-brain barrier. Once it has crossed the barrier, it is quickly converted into glutamate, which is, in turn, synthesized into the major neurotransmitter gamma-aminobutyric acid (GABA). Recommended daily amount of L-glutamine is 1,000 mg.

***Phosphatidyl Choline (Lecithin):** Acetylcholine is also a major neurotransmitter that mediates our emotions and behavior. Lecithin (phosphatidyl choline) is the richest source of choline, which is converted into acetylcholine in the brain. Recommended daily amount of lecithin is between 2,400 and 3,600 mg.

## C. A steady source of energy for optimal brain function.
The brain is unique, the most complex organ in the body. It represents only 2 percent of total body weight but accounts

for 25 percent of its oxygen utilization and consumes 70 percent of its glucose consumption. Even with such huge energy consumption, it does not have its own storage for continual energy supply. It relies solely on a constant flow of blood to supply glucose, oxygen, and other nutrients. L-glutamine can also serve as "fuel" for the brain. It is the only chemical besides glucose that can be used by the brain for energy. L-carnitine and acetyl-L-carnitine are naturally occurring nonessential amino acids that transport fats across cell membranes into the mitochondria for energy burning.

*Glucose:** Glucose is so important for human life, because it powers the brain. The brain stores so little glucose for energy production that, if not replenished, it would be all used up in less than ten minutes. If the brain cells cannot find enough or cannot properly handle the glucose, the ultimate result could be a disturbance in memory or mood. For optimal brain function, you need to maintain normal blood glucose levels. Extra high or low blood glucose levels compromise mental function. Persistent high levels of glucose from eating a high glycemic index diet can result in degradation of memory and mental functioning and make your body, including your brain, age faster by accelerating the aging process through chemical reactions in cells. This excess glucose reacts with proteins to form so-called "glycated" or "cross-linked" proteins, a kind of cellular debris that accumulates in cells. These sugar-damaged proteins are also called advanced glycosylation end products (AGEs), which are the first step that leads to diabetic nerve damage, known as neuropathy, and possibly even to age-related memory loss and some neurodegenerative diseases. For the sake of your brain health, keep your blood glucose at normal levels, and choose low glycemic carbohydrates that gradually raise blood glucose, making it steadily available to your brain.

**\*L-glutamine:** L-glutamine's major function is that it serves as "fuel" for the brain. In fact, L-glutamine is the only chemical besides glucose that can be used by the brain for energy. Now recognized as an important nutrient for the health of the brain, it can readily cross the blood-brain barrier. Research shows it could improve intelligence and help control alcoholism, schizophrenia, and a craving for sweets. A study reported that nine out of ten alcoholics after taking L-glutamine supplements had less desire to drink, less anxiety, and slept better, as compared to the placebo group, which did not do well. There are also reports that patients with bone marrow transplant were statistically more vigorous and less fatigued after taking L-glutamine. In a study reported in the *American Journal of Clinical Nutrition* in 1995 (vol. 61: 1058–61), scientists gave two grams of L-glutamine to healthy athletes and noticed that their blood levels of human growth hormone rose 430 percent above initial levels ninety minutes after supplementation. These reports demonstrated that using proper nutritional means could also help resolve neurologic problems and improve brain health. To promote your brain health, you can purchase pure L-glutamine powder (an odorless, tasteless white powder), and stir one teaspoon of this powder into your protein shake or juice, or take a 1,000 mg capsule daily.

**\*L-Carnitine and Acetyl-L-Carnitine (ALC):** L-carnitine and ALC are naturally occurring nonessential amino acids, and close relatives. They transport fats across the cell membrane into the energy-producing mitochondria of each cell. They play a critical role in maintaining youthful cellular energy, cell metabolism, and blood flow, thus protecting neurologic function from aging. ALC had been studied for many years for its effects on cognitive disorders. It appears very promising as a cognition enhancer for healthy people and as a form of treatment for age-related memory impairment. Italian researchers evaluated 236 mentally impaired elderly people who were treated with 1,500 mg of ALC a day. Those who took ALC improved significantly in memory, constructional thinking, and emotional state, as compared to the placebo group (Mcfarland, J. L., *Living without Growing Old*. Siloam Press, 2004). Researchers also studied the effects of ALC on sixty depressed patients between the ages of sixty and eighty. ALC reduced the severity of depression and improved the quality of life significantly (*International Journal of Clinical Pharmacology Research* 10.6: 355-60, 1990). Studies have also shown significant improvement and effectiveness of ALC on people with senility. Recommended daily amount is 1,000 to 2,000 mg in two divided doses.

**D. Sufficient DHA (docosahexaenoic acid) to build better brains.** The brain is the body's fattiest organ, consisting of 60 percent fats, but it has no fatty tissue reserve for energy supply or future use. The biochemistry of these fats profoundly influences the very architecture of brain cells, especially the profusion or scarcity of dendrites and synapses. As we now know, neurons can grow and expand at all ages, and such growth requires continuous supplies of fatty acids. Therefore, the fat you eat throughout life is constantly remodeling your brain.

DHA is considered to be the king of brain fats. It is a long-chain, omega-3 fatty acid, the most powerful player in brain biochemistry. It is the main structural fatty acid in the gray matter of the brain and retina of the eye. DHA is concentrated in the cell membranes of synaptic communication centers, the mitochondria of neurons, and in the photoreceptors of the eye retina. Although your body can convert plant-derived omega-3 fatty acid (short chain) to a limited amount of DHA omega-3 fatty acid, it's virtually impossible to make enough DHA to meet your brain's need through the average American diet. This is the reason why we must continually supply our brain cells with already-formed DHA by eating omega-3-rich seafood or fish oil soft gels. We need long-chain, marine omega-3 fatty acids to build strong brains and to make them operate at top condition for a lifetime. DHA alters brain cell structure and the ability of signals to get through with high-powered transmission.

Dietary fat has significant effects on brain function and helps manipulate extremely complex cognitive behavior. Research demonstrates that the more saturated fats animals eat, the more severe their brain malfunction. Analysis at the University of Waterloo, Ontario, Canada, of the effects of saturated fat on the morphology of the brain cells demonstrated that the gray matter of fat-fed animals showed fewer and shorter dendrites, with fewer of the branches needed to reach out to send and receive signals. A study by Richard Mayeux and colleagues at Columbia University showed that people over age sixty-five who ate the most saturated fat were five times more likely to develop Parkinson's disease than those who ate the least saturated fat (Carper, J., *Your Miracle Brain*. Harper-Collins, 2000).

Although omega-6 polyunsaturated fats are also essential fatty acids, needed to build cell membranes, constant and overabundant consumption of omega-6 in the average American diet creates havoc in the brain. One of the results is persistent inflammation of brain tissue, since excess omega-6s are used by the body to synthesize series 2 prostaglandins (PGE-2s), which play a role in inflammation. Such inflammation can injure cerebral blood vessels; warp nerve cell membranes, causing disruption in normal functioning; and interfere with neuronal message transmission. Furthermore, omega-6s are more rigid molecules in the cell membranes, while DHA omega-3s are fluid. A neuron that is high in DHA omega-3 is virtually liquid, allowing for more effective reception of serotonin, dopamine, and other neurotransmitters. Too many omega-6s, with their rigid molecules, in the cell membranes of neurons will adversely affect brain function. Research has demonstrated that seniors with diets high in omega-6s had poorer mental function and more memory loss.

What is most important for brain function is not only the total amount of fatty acids you eat but the relative amounts of each. Americans consume far too much omega-6 fatty acids and are deficient in marine omega-3 fatty acids. As discussed in chapter 3, the ratio of omega-6 to omega-3 fatty acids obtained through the average American diet is more like 20:1, while the ideal healthy ratio is 2:1. It has now become clear: the ratio of fatty acids you eat is the critical factor that determines how well information is transmitted from neuron to neuron.

2.  **Control of Free radical Attacks Through Wise Use of Antioxidants.** The brain, which consists of 60 percent fat, is uniquely vulnerable to oxidative injuries from increased free radical attacks and oxidative stress. This is considered to be the result of the brain's high metabolic rate. The brain generates more free radicals than other body tissues, as well as elevated levels of polyunsaturated fats (including omega-3 and omega-6 fatty acids), which are the targets of lipid peroxidation. These free radical attacks become the primary root cause of disease that damages the brain. In nerve cells, free radical attacks cause

dendrites to retract and synapses to vanish, dramatically cutting back on the nerve cells' ability to communicate. Eventually, free radical damage threatens the survival of nerve cells. The longer you live, the more free radicals are generated in the brain, making you more susceptible to age-related cognitive decline, as well as neurodegenerative diseases.

The amount of cumulative damage and cognitive decline depends greatly on the strength of your antioxidant defenses to control free radical attacks. Unfortunately, the production of endogenous antioxidants, such as superoxide dismutase (SOD), alpha lipoic acid, and coenzyme Q10, is greatly reduced in seniors; thus, a steady supply of proper antioxidant supplements in addition to eating antioxidant-rich fruits and vegetables to protect your brain is all-important in seniors, especially those with food digestion and absorption problems. The following antioxidant supplements are recommended for seniors:

> **\*Red Wine with Onion:** This do-it-yourself, "enhanced" red wine recipe, provided in chapter 6 and at the back of the book, is a heart health-promoting and cancer risk-reducing combination that is also good for brain health. Red wine contains resveratrol and is exceptionally high in the antioxidant polyphenol, particularly anthocyanins. In addition, onion is high in the antioxidant quercetin. Alcohol itself has anti-inflammatory effects. This is important because inflammation in the brain contributes to blood vessel and nerve cell destruction and possibly Alzheimer's disease. New evidence suggests that alcohol blocks AGE formation by inhibiting the damaging protein-sugar reactions in nerve cells that accelerate cell aging, memory decline, and poor mental functioning. One study at the Indiana University School of Medicine found that elderly light drinkers (fewer

than four drinks per week) scored better on cognitive tests than nondrinkers. But those who drank ten or more drinks per week scored poorly. A French study of 3,700 French men and women over age sixty-five found that moderate drinkers of red wine were only 18 percent as likely as nondrinkers to suffer severe intellectual decline with age and only 25 percent as apt to develop Alzheimer's disease (Carper, J., *Your Miracle Brain.* Harper, 2000).

**\*Alpha Lipoic Acid:** Alpha lipoic acid is considered to be the most versatile and powerful of all antioxidants. It has the unique ability to be rapidly absorbed from the gut, and it readily crosses the blood-brain barrier because of its small molecules. After entering the central nervous system, it is quickly taken up by brain tissue and goes directly to rescue the nerve cells under attack. Unlike any other antioxidant, it is both water- and fat-soluble and thus able to exert its action in both fluid (cytoplasm) and fatty (membrane) portions of the cells. It can also neutralize the very type of free radical, the nitrogen free radical, that is particularly hazardous to nerve cells. With age, energy production in mitochondria declines, meaning that they utilize oxygen and glucose less efficiently and produce more free radical damage. Alpha lipoic acid is able to increase the efficiency of energy production of the mitochondria. German researchers at the Clinical Institute for Mental Health in Mannheim showed that alpha lipoic acid may restore youthful memory and suggested that its antioxidant activity drastically slowed brain deterioration by preventing neuron losses and/or repairing faulty neuronal transmission systems. In diabetics, high blood sugar and insulin levels can attack and destroy nerve cells, known as diabetic neuropathy. Alpha lipoic acid has been used successfully to treat this condition for more than thirty years in Europe. German investigators have demonstrated that alpha lipoic acid can even stimulate regeneration of nerve fibers in those patients with diabetic neuropathy. Lester Packer, professor of molecular and cell biology, University of California at Berkeley and one of the world's leading researchers on antioxidants, suggests that alpha lipoic acid can be used to prevent the onset of type II diabetes by helping stabilize blood sugar and insulin levels (*Free Radical Biology and Medicine*, 20:625-26, 1996). Recommended daily amount is 100 to 200 mg—if you are diabetic, 200 to 600 mg. No toxic effects have been reported, even in high doses.

**\*Coenzyme Q10 (CoQ10):** CoQ10 is a brain booster and rejuvenator, helping protect your brain against aging and the accompanying cognitive decline. It is fat-soluble and works in the fatty membranes of nerve cells, where the potential for damage by lipid peroxidation is greatest. In fact, lipid peroxidation is the key reason why nerve cells disintegrate, malfunction, and may even be destroyed. Lipid peroxidation is just the initial stage of the beginning of the end of a nerve cell. A brain without adequate CoQ10 cannot work at full power, so memory and learning abilities decline, and the brain becomes more vulnerable to age-related neurodegenerative diseases. Since CoQ10 levels drop as you age, taking a CoQ10 supplement is necessary to rejuvenate brain cells. In patients with Parkinson's disease, CoQ10 levels were found to be exceptionally low. Researchers have also discovered that Parkinson's disease involves two defects that CoQ10 is good at fixing. One is a dysfunction in the mitochondria's energy production. Another is the free radical damage to nerve cells in a part of the brain called the substantia nigra that produces dopamine. CoQ10 looks very promising in preventing and treating Parkinson's disease (Carper, J., *Your Miracle Brain*. Harper-Collins, 2000). Recommended daily amount is 100 to 300 mg for seniors. Those who are taking cholesterol-lowering drugs, which tend to deplete reserves of CoQ10, need be sure they also take ample CoQ10 supplements.

**\*Melatonin:** Melatonin is made from tryptophan, an essential amino acid, meaning that we must get the raw material from the foods we eat or supplements we take in order to make this hormone. Our body converts tryptophan into serotonin; then, at night, serotonin is converted in the pineal gland into melatonin. The initial clinical studies on melatonin focused on problems related to the sleep-wake cycle. Now we understand that melatonin is an important hormone that stimulates the release of a wide variety of other hormones from the pituitary gland during sleep. Russell Reiter, PhD, after researching melatonin for more than thirty years, has concluded that melatonin is the most powerful antioxidant molecule yet to be discovered (*Journal of Pineal Research*, 18: 1–11, 1995). It plays an important role in protecting brain health. Melatonin can inhibit the action of free radicals and can even blunt the destructive effects of cortisol, the stress hormone that may cause neuronal dendrites to shrivel up and nerve cells responsible for memory to die after weeks or months of exposure to elevated levels. It has been shown to protect against a variety of degenerative and age-related neurological conditions of the brain, such as Parkinson's disease, schizophrenia, and depression. The pineal gland secretes melatonin during times of darkness, and secretion is suppressed by bright light. Adequate amounts of melatonin induce sleep and may reduce anxiety, panic disorders, and migraines. Recommended daily dosage for seniors is 3 to 5 mg at bedtime. There are no known side effects.

3. **Lifestyle Changes.** We have considerable control over our later years. For most of us, our long-term quality of life is driven mainly by the eating habits and lifestyle choices we make today. Only a small portion of the characteristics of aging is genetically based, meaning that we seniors are largely responsible for our own old age. Lifestyle choice is certainly a powerful determinant of mental functioning during the process of aging.

   *\*Drink alcohol only in moderation:* Studies find that too much alcohol can damage the brain. Heavy drinking of any alcoholic beverage can kill brain cells, leading to brain atrophy, decline in cognitive functions, and dementia. One study at the Indiana University School of Medicine found that seniors who drank ten or more drinks per week scored more poorly on cognitive tests than nondrinkers.

   *\*No smoking:* Cigarette smoking impairs pulmonary and cardiac functions, reduces the supply of oxygen and nutrients to your brain, and leads to cognitive decline.

   *\*Practice stress reduction:* Stress has prompted unhealthy behaviors, such as alcohol abuse, smoking, and sleep deprivation, and it can even cause brain damage. Common sources among seniors include job strain, daily hurried pace, family problems, and financial worries. Research reveals that persistent stress can alter both the structure and functioning of the brain cells. High levels of the stress hormone cortisol can reduce axon sprouting and dendrite branching, both of which underlie learning and memory.

   *\*Stay mentally active:* Research has produced evidence that the way you use your brain can alter its structure. Stimulating your brain intellectually can prod the brain to produce new connections between neurons and even create new brain cells. Consistent mental stimulation actually builds more

brain tissue, giving you a "bigger memory board." Thus, education makes brains more resistant to deterioration and dementia as you age.

**\*Remain physically active:** Several studies find that physical exercise has a beneficial effect on the brains of the elderly, mainly because it improves blood flow to the brain. Research also showed that exercise might even spur growth of dendrites not only in parts of the brain controlling motor function, but also in areas controlling memory, reasoning, thinking, and learning.

**\*Don't use illegal drugs:** Illegal drugs may reduce the production of some neurotransmitters and deplete their reserves, which, in turn, slow down the neuronal message transmission. Furthermore, neurotransmitters may be blocked from reaching their proper receptors as a result of using certain drugs. The malfunction of neurotransmitters then results in neurological problems.

We can see that several risk factors are involved in the loss of cognitive ability in seniors. Because of the uniqueness and complexity of brain physiology, biochemistry, pathology, and nutritional needs, any one measure, one drug, or a few supplements does not guarantee a total protective effect against age-related declines in brain function. There is a great deal we can do naturally and nutritionally to enhance the health of the brain. We can reduce risks for mental deterioration and cognitive decline, and, possibly, a host of chronic neurodegenerative diseases. First, with a healthy cardiovascular system and proper supplementation of essential and special nutrients, the human brain is able to manufacture the needed quantity of neurotransmitters for optimal brain function. Second, with a steady supply of proper antioxidant supplements, in addition to antioxidant-rich fruits and vegetables, your brain cells are synergistically protected from destruction. Third, by choosing good habits over bad, you can reduce the risk of cognitive decline in the aging process. After all, we seniors are largely responsible for the quality of life in our own old age. A readiness to change and a positive mindset are keys to success. The first step is to set a goal. A small attainable goal encourages success. It's never too late to improve your brain health. Let your whole body work synergistically to increase the chances of success.

# Chapter 10
# Taking Charge of Your Own Health:
# Maintaining Quality of Life

Every human body begins life as a single cell, a fertilized ovum. By adulthood, the human body consists of 100 trillion cells, which are the fundamental components of all living things. As cells deteriorate, people age. As cells malfunction, people get sick. Every living cell in your body is mainly composed of protein. The body must have a continuous supply of protein to sustain life. Each gene in the chromosome of your cells possesses codes for a protein and can instruct the body to construct a particular protein out of the amino acids absorbed by the intestinal tract after the digestion of the protein that we eat. Some proteins are long-lived, others short-lived. In those cells that make up our supporting framework (such as bones, muscles, and cartilages), the proteins are long-lived and do not turn over frequently. The proteins that make up our vital organs are short-lived and are replaced more frequently. The various cells, whether made up of long- or short-lived proteins, can only replicate a limited number of times. When the cells fail to replicate, we eventually age and die.

Scientists have found that our chromosomes have small caps on the ends, called *telomeres*, that control cell replication. Every time a cell reproduces, that telomere gets a little shorter. Telomere shortening appears to be a key part of cellular aging. In multiple studies, short telomere length in white blood cells has been shown to predict death, cardiovascular events, and heart failure. We need a substance called *telomerase* to rebuild the ends of the chromosomes to keep cells healthy. Telomerase is overactive in 85 percent of cancers, allowing cancer cells to reproduce and spread faster than normal cells. The amount of telomerase a person has depends on genetics, but it can be influenced and adjusted by lifestyle changes and nutritional modification. However, many cells in our body don't have telomerase, meaning that those cells have a reproduction limit. People with chronic stress have shortened telomeres, meaning that cell replication is limited.

New research found that marine omega-3 fatty acids were associated with decelerated telomere attrition over five years, and heart patients with high omega-3 fatty acid intake had relatively longer telomeres (Oz, M. C., and Roizen, M. F., *Staying Young*. Free Press, 2007). Cardiologists from the University of California, San Francisco, and other hospitals measured telomere length over five years in 608 patients who had coronary-artery blockage and previous heart attacks. They found that patients with high blood levels of omega-3 fatty acids experienced significantly less shortening of telomeres as well as markedly reduced subsequent cardiac and all-cause mortality over five years, as compared with patients with lower omega-3 levels (*Journal of American Medical Association*, November 2010). This result appears to demonstrate a new link between omega-3 fatty acids, which modify telomeres, and the aging process. It also implies that telomere length can be a predictor of risk of mortality in humans.

Researchers are now also focusing on a longevity gene present in almost all life forms: the sirtuin gene. It's normally inactive, but when it is active, it triggers a survival mechanism that extends life. Resveratrol is a sirtuin gene stimulator and in studies on mice has been found to prevent or slow the progression of illnesses from cancer to cardiovascular disease. It has even extended the life span of laboratory specimens, including yeast, flies, worms, and mice (*Molecular Endocrinology*, August 2007). However, results in laboratory animal studies are not always applicable to the human body. The human body is a lot more complicated than the bodies of lab animals, and many human body functions are under the influence of the central nervous system, which is rather rudimentary in lab animals.

It appears that the human body's aging rate is partly genetically driven, but it can be significantly modified by environment, nutrition, and lifestyle-related choices. While genes are certainly an important component of the aging process, they may not be the most relevant factor, meaning that the majority of other variables are in our hands.

Aging is a systemic process: it affects not only specific areas of the body but the body as a whole. Dysfunction in one area is often echoed in other areas. The aging rates of the bodily systems vary considerably from person to person. No one can turn back the aging clock, but we certainly can ameliorate many of the effects commonly associated with aging. For instance, healthy heart muscle is rarely weakened by increasing age alone, but it is greatly weakened by vascular disease, which can be prevented by making healthy lifestyle and nutrition choices. There is a great deal we can do naturally and nutritionally to enhance the health of the heart and to prevent instances of heart disease. The following lifestyle and nutrition factors have positive impacts on heart health:

- Normal body weight maintenance

- Regular physical exercise

- Stress relief

- Smoke-free environment

- Lower sugar and salt consumption

- Proper diet with more foods of plant origin and limited intake of red meat

- Elimination of hydrogenated or hardened fats

- Limited consumption of alcohol

- Proper vitamin and mineral intake

- Adequate antioxidants

- Normal homocysteine blood level maintenance from taking folic acid and vitamin B-12

Senility is not inevitable as age advances. Everybody ages, but only some become senile. Memory deterioration or even loss, inability to store new information, and certain personality quirks associated with senility can be postponed, if not prevented. Just as senility is not inevitable, neither are most chronic degenerative diseases. A person can age without many of the age-related diseases that we have come to assume are inescapable. It is certainly possible that we can slow down the aging process and in many instances prevent physical and mental degeneration. From my own experience I am convinced that chronic degenerative disease is not an inevitable part of aging process, and it is certainly possible for us to not only live a long life, but to be energetic and healthy.

The Center for Disease Control has stated that in this country 54 percent of heart disease, 37 percent of cancer, 50 percent of cerebrovascular disease, and 49 percent of atherosclerosis is preventable through lifestyle and diet modification. That means some 1.6 million deaths a year can be prevented, and there is a great hope for people willing to take charge of their health. Many people are aging too rapidly and dying from conditions that can be prevented. There is a great deal you can do to support your health and prevent premature death. That's what this book intends to help you accomplish.

The causes of many chronic degenerative diseases are often associated with either the absence or deficiency of one or more chemical substances in your system or too much of other chemical substances. This occurs even when you think you are on a proper healthy diet. Those chemical substances, in many instances related to nutrition, are nearly always something you can add to or delete from your body. You need to learn how to take charge of your health through dietary modifications and wise use of nutritional supplementation. By doing so, you may eliminate some unnecessary medications.

No two individuals have the same genetic makeup, hormonal balance, or cellular structures. Despite our individual differences, one goal is shared by all of us: the goal of achieving optimal health. Good health is far more than the simple absence of disease. If you are healthy, your body is always trying to make you feel well. It is constantly in the process of making trillions of new cells. These cells have to harvest your bloodstream or tissue fluids for sustenance that consists of eight essential and two semi-essential amino acids, thirteen vitamins, sixteen essential minerals and trace elements, two essential fatty acids, and various enzymes, all of which are crucial to sustain life but not manufactured by your body. These chemical substances must come from the food we eat and the water we drink. When the food is cured, processed, hydrogenated, preserved, refined, emulsified, bleached, colorized, and sterilized, something is lost. In many instances, it is our health that is lost. Recognizing subtle deviations from good health and taking steps to correct them early is preventive medicine at its best.

Baby boomers as well as current senior citizens want to age without growing feeble and sick. You can retain an attractive appearance and vitality while you pile on calendar years. However, health is not something that just happens. Make a decision today that you are going to strive for optimal health and that you are going to become healthy through natural and nutritional means. You can take charge of your health and slow down the aging process through this whole-body approach.

To implement this approach, first you need to bring your body back to optimal physiological condition, with a healthy pH of 7.4 in both intracellular and extracellular tissue fluids, where most physiological functions take place, mainly by enzymatic reactions. Enzymatic reactions can complete their task correctly and efficiently only in an environment with a clearly defined pH. By restoring the acid-alkaline balance in the tissue fluids to this slightly alkaline pH of 7.4, the human body conducts optimal physiological functions, including metabolism, tissue repair, enzymatic reactions, and immune function.

Second, you need to learn to boost your immune system through natural and nutritional means. A fully functioning immune system can protect you by eliminating foreign invaders and internal precancerous dysplastic cells, as well as by tightly regulating the inflammatory response in tissues.

Third, you also need to effectively control free radical attacks, which are genuine troublemakers. They are abundant and endogenous, both intracellular or extracellular. Wise use of antioxidants can help you put an end to their destructive damage to cells and tissues.

You are now on the road to better health. By allowing the whole body to work together synergistically to protect your health and increase the chance of success, you will always be one step ahead in preventing or treating various health problems in a whole-body perspective. This approach is designed to treat various health problems that have not yet shown up but are possibly in the making. This is preventive medicine at its best.

The most important investment you can make in your senior years is the investment in your health. Too many people are aging too rapidly and are succumbing to illnesses that are preventable. Although this investment involves lifestyle and diet modification, their benefits come in spades. I was able to do it, and I am sure that you can do it too. My experience tells me that disease is not an inevitable part of aging. It is possible for us to not only live longer lives, but to live them in disease-free, healthier bodies. You must take charge of your health, because no one else is going to do it for you. These health benefits will be valuable many years into your future. Your face, body, and energy level are constant visible monitors of how well or how poorly you are aging. Looking good and having a healthy and energetic body during a long and happy life is not wishful thinking; it is your goal.

For the time being, the longer life expectancy in this country is accompanied by increased disability from cardiovascular disease, osteoporosis, age-related cancer, and loss of cognitive ability among seniors. As a result, the need for services and care from health facilities is growing more urgent. At the same time, the government is struggling to deal with skyrocketing healthcare costs and to provide coverage for the whole population. It is my wish that my own experience can inspire seniors to improve their health through natural and nutritional means. Preventive medicine requires a multifaceted approach: proper diet with necessary supplements, regular physical and mental exercises, and changes in improper eating habits and lifestyle. All these measures work synergistically to gradually bring your body back to optimal physiological condition with a fully functioning immune system, thereby putting you on the road to better health. These approaches will not only bring about personal well-being but untold savings in medical treatments. With an ever-increasing population of well-informed individuals motivated to safeguard their own health, the day may come when healthcare is indeed healthcare and not the "disease-care" we have nowadays.

# 1. My Recipe for Reducing the Risks of Age-Related Diseases

(Liang-Che Tao, MD)

A. **Before Breakfast**

    1. Fish Oil: DHA and EPA, 1,000 mg

    2. Lecithin: 2,400 mg

    3. CoQ10: 200 mg

    4. Alpha Lipoic Acid: 200 mg

    5. Resveratrol: 250 mg

B. **During Breakfast**

    1. Freshly-squeezed vegetable and fruit juice: 200 ml

C. **During Lunch**

    1. Red wine with onion *: 100 ml

    2. Pure pomegranate juice: 8 oz

D. **After Lunch**

    1. Multivitamin pill

    2. Magnesium: 400 mg

    3. Folic Acid: 400 mcg

E. **Before Bedtime**

    1. Melatonin: 3 mg

    2. L- Tryptophan: 500 mg

    3. L-Tyrosine: 500 mg

    4. L-Carnitine: 1,000 mg

## 2. Recipe for Red Wine with Onion:

One large yellow onion (2 cups when chopped)

750 ml red wine

Cut the onion into small pieces, and set aside for 10 minutes. Do not rinse the cut onion, so as to preserve the water-soluble quercetin. Into a decanter, combine 750 ml red wine and the cut onion, and let soak for 10 days. Pour the onion wine through a filter, and discard the onion.

# Suggested Reading

Beliveau, R. and Gingras, D. *Foods That Fight Cancer: Preventing Cancer through Diet.* Toronto: McClelland & Stewart, 2006.

Benton, D. *Food for Thought.* London: Penguin Books, 1996.

Blaylock, R. L. *Excitotoxins: The Taste that Kills.* Santa Fe: Health Press, 1997.

Bloomfield, H. H. *Hypericum and Depression.* Los Angeles: Prelude Press, 1996.

Booth, W. *The Art of Growing Older: Writers on Living and Aging.* Chicago: University of Chicago Press, 1996.

Brand-Miller, J., and Wolever, J. *The Glucose Revolution.* New York: Marlowe & Company, 1999.

Brown, D. J. *Herbal Prescriptions for Better Health.* Rocklin, California: Prima Publishing, 1996.

Brown, R., Bottiglieri, T, and Colman, C. *Stop Depression Now.* New York: G.P. Putnam & Sons, 1999.

Carper, J. *Stop Aging Now!* New York: Harper-Collins, 1996.

Carper, J. *Miracle Cures.* New York: Harper-Collins, 1998.

Carper, J. *Your Miracle Brain.* New York: Harper-Collins, 2000.

Christensen, L. *Diet-Behavior Relationships*. Washington, D.C.: American Psychological Association, 1996.

Crook, T. H., and Adderly, B. *The Memory Cure*. New York: Pocket Books,1998.

Diamond, M., and Hopson, J. *Magic Trees of the Mind: How to Nurture Your Child's Intelligence, Creativity and Healthy Emotions*. New York: Dutton,1998.

Duke, J. A. *The Green Pharmacy*. Emmaus, Pennsylvania: Rodale Press, 1997.

Dychtwald, K. *Age Power: How the 21$^{st}$ Century Will Be Ruled by the New Old*. Los Angeles: Tarcher, 2000.

Fugh-Berman, A. *Alternative Medicine: What Works*. Tucson, Arizona: Odonian Press, 1996.

Gordon, J. S. *Manifesto for a New Medicine*. Reading, Massachusetts: Addison-Wesley Publishing Company, 1996.

Harman, D., Hollidays, R., and Meydani, M. "Towards Prolongation of the Healthy Life Span." *Annals of the New York Academy of Sciences*, Volume 854, 1998.

Hayflick, L. *How and Why We Age*. New York: Ballantine, 1996.

Heber, D. *What Color Is Your Diet?* New York: Regan Books, 2002.

Holstein, L. *How to Have Magnificent Sex: Improve Your Relationship and Start to Have the Best Sex of Your Life*. New York: Three Rivers Press, 2003.

Kirkwood, T. *The Time of Our Lives: The Science of Human Aging*. New York: Oxford University Press, 1999.

Kotulak, R. *Inside the Brain: Revolutionary Discoveries of How the Mind Works*. Kansas City: Andrews McMeel Publishing, 1996.

Lane, N. *Oxygen: The Molecule That Made the World*. New York: Oxford University Press, 2002.

Lanou, A. J., and Castleman, M. *Building Bone Vitality: A Revolutionary Diet Plan to Prevent Bone Loss and Reverse Osteoporosis*. New York: McGraw-Hill, 2009.

Lombard, J., and Germano, C. *The Brain Wellness Plan*. New York: Kensington, 1997.

Mahoney, D., and Restak, R. *Longevity Strategy: How to Live to 100 Using the Brain-Body Connection*. New Jersey: Wiley, 1999.

Mccormick, R. K. *The Whole-Body Approach to Osteoporosis: How to Improve Bone Strength and Reduce Your Fracture Risk*. Oakland: New Harbinger Publications, 2009.

McFarland, J. L. *Aging without Growing Old*. Lake Mary: Siloam Press, 2004.

Murray, M. T. *Encyclopedia of Nutritional Supplements*. Rocklin, California: Prima Publishing, 1996.

Olshansky, S. J., and Carnes, B. *The Quest for Immortality: Science at the Frontiers of Aging*. New York: W.W. Norton, 2001.

Oz, M. C., and Roizen, M. F. *Staying Young: The Owner's Manual to Extending Your Warranty*. New York: Free Press, 2007.

Packer, L. *The Antioxidant Miracle*. New York: John Wiley & Sons, Inc. 1999.

Packer, L., Hiramatsu, M., and Yoshikawa, T. *Free Radicals in Brain Physiology and Disorders*. San Diego: Academic Press, 1996.

Papas, A. *The Vitamin E Revolution.* New York: Harper-Collins, 1999.

Perlmutter, D., and Colman, C. *The Better Brain Book: The Best Tools for Improving Memory and Sharpness and for Preventing Aging of the Brain.* New York: Riverhead Books, 2004.

Perls, T. T., Silver, M. H., and Lauerman, J. *Living to 100: Lessons in Living to Your Maximum Potential at Any Age.* New York: Basic Books, 2000.

Perricone, N. *The Perricone Prescription: A Physician's 28-day Program for Total Body and Face Rejuvenation.* New York: Harper Resource, 2002.

Perricone, N. *The Perricone Promise: Look Younger, Live Longer in Three Easy Steps.* New York: Warner Books, 2004.

Pizzorno, J. *Total Wellness.* Rocklin, California: Prima Publishing, 1996.

Roizen, M. *The Real Age Makeover: Take Years off Your Looks and Add Them to Your Life.* New York: Harper-Collins, 2004.

Rose, M. *The Long Tomorrow: How Evolution Can Help Us Postpone Aging.* New York: Oxford University Press, 2005.

Rosenthal, N. *St. John's Wort.* New York: Harper-Collins, 1998.

Rowe, J. W., and Kahn, R. L. *Successful Aging.* New York: Pantheon, 1998.

Sapolsky, R. M. *Why Zebras Don't Get Ulcers: An updated guide to stress, stress-related diseases, and coping, 2nd ed.* New York: W. H. Freeman, 1998.

Schachter-Shalomi, Z., and Miller, R. S. *From Age-ing to Sage-ing: A Profound New Vision of Growing Older.* New York: Warner Books, 1997.

Schmidt, M. A. *Smart Fats*. Berkeley: Frog Ltd, 1997.

Servan-Schrieber, D. *Anticancer: A New Way of Life*. London: Viking, 2008.

Sinatra, S. T. *Optimum Health*. New York: Bantam Books, 1997.

Snowdon, D. *Aging with Grace: What the Nun Study Teaches Us about Leading Longer, Healthier, and More Meaningful Lives*. New York: Bantam, 2002.

Theodosakis, J., Brenda, A., and Barry, F. *The Arthritis Cure*. New York: St. Martin's Press, 1997.

Vaillant, G. E. *Aging Well: Surprising Guideposts to a Happier Life from the Landmark Harvard Study of Adult Development*. Boston: Little, Brown, 2003.

Weil, A. *Eating Well for Optimum Health: The Essential Guide to Bringing Health and Pleasure Back to Eating*. New York: Harper-Collins, 2001.

Weil, A. *Eight Weeks to Optimum Health: A Proven Program for Taking Full Advantage of Your Body's Natural Healing Power, Rev. ed.* New York: Ballantine, 2006.

Weil, A. *Healthy Aging: A Lifelong Guide to Your Well-Being*. New York: Random House, 2005.

Weil, A. *Natural Health, Natural Medicine: The Complete Guide to Wellness and Self-Care for Optimum Health, Rev. ed.* Boston: Houghton Mifflin, 2004.

Weil, A. *Spontaneous Healing: How to Discover and Embrace Your Body's Natural Ability to Maintain and Heal Itself*. New York: Ballantine Books, 2000.

Willcox, B. J., Willcox, D. C., and Suzuki, M. *The Okinawa Program: How the World's Longest-Lived People Achieve Everlasting Health—and How You Can Too*. New York: Three Rivers Press, 2002.

Willett, W., and Skerrett, P. J. *Eat, Drink, and Be Healthy: The Harvard Medical School Guide to Healthy Eating*. New York: Free Press, 2002.

Woodruff-Pak, D. S. *The Neuropsychology of Aging*. Malden, MA: Blackwell Publishers, Inc., 1997.

Yee, R. *Moving Toward Balance: 8 Weeks of Yoga with Rodney Yee*. Emmaus, PA: Rodale Press, 2004.

# Index

beta blockers, 53
beta-carotene, 61, 63, 64, 92
Beta-Carotene and Retinol Trial, 61
beverages, 16, 17, 43, 89, 104. *See also*
    coffee; juice; soft drinks; tea
bioelectrical impedance analysis (BIA),
    3
bioflavonoids, 64, 65
biopsy, 113
birth defects, 139
bispheol A (BPA), 23–24
bladder cancer, 111, 115
bladder stones, 105
Blocadren, 53
blood, pH level of, 2
blood cholesterol levels,35, 78, 80,
    83, 84, 86. *See also* high-density
    lipoprotein (HDL) cholesterol; low-
    density lipoprotein (LDL) cholesterol
blood clot formation, 21, 27, 28,35, 49,
    74, 81–82, 83, 90, 100, 118
blood glucose, 7, 37, 54, 142
blood glucose-lowering drugs, 54–55.
    *See also specific medications*
blood pressure-lowering drugs, 53–54.
    *See also specific medications*
blood tests, 113
Blucotrol, 54
BMD (bone mineral density), 102
body fluids
    analysis of, 3
    pH of, 2
body weight, 3, 78, 127, 141, 157
bone density-enhancing drugs, 51–52.
    *See also specific medications*
bone formation, 98, 103, 106, 109
bone fractures, 52, 99, 103. *See also* hip
    fractures
bone mineral density (BMD), 102
bone mineral density T score, 99
bone remodeling, 107
bone resorption, 5, 98, 102, 103, 109
Boniva, 51, 52
boron, 20, 40, 41, 105–106
BPA (bispheol A), 23–24

brain. *See also* cognitive ability
    and cholesterol, 78
    described, 127–129, 134, 141–142
    and DHA, 21,35
    fat content of,34
    and free radical attacks, 8, 60
brain function, age-related decline in,
    129, 131
brain shrinkage, 134, 135
breast cancer, 4, 24, 66, 72, 74, 111,
    112, 118–119, 121
*British Journal of Cancer*, 66
broccoli, 64, 65, 101, 122
Brussel sprouts, 68, 122
buckwheat, 65
*Building Bone Vitality* (Lanou and
    Castleman), 99, 102, 167
burning sensation, 48, 139
*Business Week*, 50

## C

cabbage, 122
caffeinated beverages, 43. *See also* coffee;
    soft drinks; tea
calcium, 6, 17, 19, 40, 42, 48, 98, 100,
    101, 102, 105
calcium carbonate, 98, 101
calcium channel blockers, 54
calcium-phosophorous ratios, 100–101
calorie restriction, 11–12, 37
Cambridge Heart Antioxidant Study, 92
*Cancer*, 112, 114
cancer
    age-related, 29,34, 111, 115,
        117–126
    described, 111
    diagnosis and prognosis of, 112–
        113
    and melatonin, 72
    occurrences of, in the world, 112
    occurrences of, in US, 112
    percent preventable, 158
    reducing risk of age-related cancer,
        117–126
    types of. *See specific cancers*

in Japan, 20
and neurotransmitter levels, 140
and phosphorous, 100, 107
proper diet with necessary
supplements, 19–22
protein in, 102, 103
raising alkalinity in tissue fluids
through, 15–16, 52, 89, 102
standard American diet, 20, 22,32,
100, 145, 146
and vitamin D, 105
diet modification, benefits of, 158–160
dietary chemicals, brain sensitivity to,
129
dietary control, of serotonin, 132
dietary fat, effect on brain function, 145
dietary guidelines, to help lower risk of
cancer, 122
dietary interventions, for cancer risk
reduction, 119
dietary protein, 102
digestive disorders, 38, 138
digestive enzymes, 13, 14, 55, 71
Dilantin, 51, 108
diphenhydramine, 55
distilled water, 43
diuretics, 41, 43, 53, 79
dizziness, 51, 53, 54, 55
DNA, 8, 25, 63, 66, 115, 116, 124,
139
docosahexaenoic acid (DHA), 21,35,
144–145, 146, 162
dopamine, 21, 132–133, 141, 146, 149
*Drug Safety*, 49
drug use, illegal, 136, 152
drug-drug interactions, 47, 56, 58
drug-induced hepatitis, 47, 49, 50, 56
drug-related deaths, 45
Dunstan, David, 17
Dymalor, 54
Dyrenium, 53
dysplastic cells, 7, 29, 113, 114, 117,
123–124, 126. *See also* precancerous
dysplastic cells

**E**

eating habits
diet. *See* diet
effects of heavy meals, 28, 86
as factor in aging, 1
and pH of blood and tissue fluids,
12
and preventive medicine, 161
and quality of life, 151
as weapons against genes, 2
edema, 138
Effexor, 51
eggs, 16,33, 63, 66, 67, 78, 102, 133
eicosapentaenoic acid (EPA), 21
emaciation,34
embolus, 82
endogenous acid products,34, 102
endogenous antioxidants, 62, 147
endogenous cholesterol,36
endometrial cancers, 121
endorphins, 132
endoscopy, 113
enery (ATP) production, 68, 93
environmental contamination, 1, 23,
115, 123
Environmental Working Group, 19
enzymatic reactions, 4, 6, 8, 25, 68,
117, 124, 160
enzymes, 6, 8, 13, 14, 18,32,33, 37, 39,
40, 49, 55, 62, 66, 159
EPA omega-3 fatty acids, 21–22,35, 90,
162
epilepsy, 138
epithelial cells, 29, 113, 114, 123
Epstein-Barr virus, 116, 123
erectile dysfunction, 51
Esidrex, 53
esophagus, 87
esophogeal cancer, 115, 121
essential amino acids, 6, 19,31,32,33,
71, 83, 90, 121, 132, 150, 159
essential fatty acids, 6, 19,31,32, 90,
121, 145, 159
essential minerals, 6, 16, 19,31,32, 40,
43, 90, 109, 121, 159

human immunodeficiency virus (HIV), 116, 117, 123
human papillomavirus, 114, 116, 121, 123
hydrochloric acid (HCl) deficiency, 139
hydrochrothiazide, 53
hydrogenated (hardened) fats,34, 158
hydroxide, 101
hyperglycemia, 82
hypertension, 49, 82, 88, 137
hypotension, 53, 54
hypothyroidism, 64
Hytrin, 53

**I**

ibuprofen, 45, 49
Icy Hot Cream, 47
IgA deficiency, 117
illegal drug use, 136, 152
immune function/system
    and acid-alkaline balance, 4, 160
    and alcohol abuse, 117, 121, 123
    being compromised, 24, 47, 56
    boosting of, 18–24
    and calcium, 100
    described,31
    deterioration of, 6–7, 119
    and DHEA, 73
    dysfunction of, 9, 117
    effect of cortisol on, 22
    and glutathione, 71
    healthful diet for optimal immune function,32–44, 90–91, 121
    and lycopene supplementation, 65
    and marine omega-3 fatty acids, 20
    and melatonin, 72, 125
    and physical exercise, 17
    and supplements, 19–22
    and vitamin A, 63
    and zinc, 66
immunoglobulin IgG, 69
immunohistochemistry, 113
immunosuppressive therapy, 117
incomplete proteins,33
Inderal, 53

Indiana University, 147, 151
Indocin, 49
infants, amount of body fluids, 3
inferior vena cava, 87
inflammation, 1–2, 18, 22, 82, 117, 145–146
inflammatory markers, 82
inflammatory response, 18,35, 89–90
information overload, ix
inhaled corticosteroids, 51, 108
insecticides, 23
insomnia, 46, 51, 55
intellectual impairment, 139
internal jugular vein, 87
*International Journal of Cancer*, 62
*International Journal of Clinical Pharmacology Research*, 144
*International Journal of Epidemiology*, 102
intracellular tissue fluid, 3, 6, 57
iodine, 17, 40
ionizing radiation, 114, 115–116, 123
iron, 6, 19, 40, 48, 56, 68, 133
Israel, cholesterol levels and rates of cardiovascular disease in, 27

**J**

jacbone necrosis, 52
Jackson, Michael, 45
*JAMA (Journal of the American Medical Association)*, 45, 51, 52, 67, 156
Japan, diets in, 20
Johns Hopkins Medical School, 74
*Journal of Clinical Endocrinology and Metabolism*, 5, 52, 102
*Journal of National Cancer Institute*, 61
*Journal of Pineal Research*, 150
*Journal of the American Dental Association*, 52
*Journal of the American Dietetic Association*, 20
*Journal of the American Geriatrics Society*,36
*Journal of the American Medical Association (JAMA)*, 45, 51, 52, 67,

156

*Journal of the National Cancer Institute*, 4, 118

juice
    pomegranate juice, 95, 162
    recommended daily intake of, 88–89, 104, 120, 162

Jupiter Trial, 50

## K

kale, 64, 65, 101, 122

Kaposi's sacroma, 116, 117

kidney cancer, 115, 119

kidney stones, 105

Klonopin, 51, 108

Kupffer cells, 24, 56

## L

*Lancet Oncology*, 115

*The Lancet*,36, 73, 84

Lanou, A. J., 99, 102, 167

Lasix, 53

L-carnitine, 26, 70, 92, 93, 142, 143–144, 162

LDL (low-density lipoprotein) cholesterol, 8, 27, 28,36, 54, 70, 79, 80, 81, 84, 91, 92, 93, 95

lecithin (phosphatidyl choline), 86, 91, 133, 141, 162

Ledger, Heath, 45

left subclavian vein, 87

legumes, 37, 38, 122

lemon, 15

lentils, 122

leucocytes, 18,31, 121

leukemia, 111

Levoxyl, 51, 108

Lexapro, 51

L-glutamine, 71, 134, 141, 142, 143

life expectancy
    and antioxidant supplements, 60–61
    changes in, in Japan, 20
    in US, 11, 26, 161

lifestyle
    changes, 83, 106–107, 119, 121, 129, 136, 151–158
    as factor in aging, 1, 2, 118
    improper lifestyle, 2, 5, 9, 136

lignin, 38

linoleic acid. *See* omega-6 (linoleic acid) fatty acids

lipid absorption, 87

lipid nutrients, 19, 85–86, 87

lipid peroxidation, 8, 60, 128, 135, 146, 149

lipid peroxides (rancid fats),34–35

lipids,34, 85

Lipitor, 50, 84

lipofuscin, 4, 69

lipoprotein lipase, 18

Lisinopril, 53

litmus paper, 14

liver (food product), 133

liver cancer, 112, 116

liver failure, 24, 46

*Living without Growing Old* (McFarland), 144

long-chain omega-3 fatty acids, 21, 22

Lopressor, 53

Lotensin, 53

Lou Gehrig's disease, 50

low blood sugar, 138

low-density lipoprotein (LDL) cholesterol, 8, 27, 28,36, 54, 70, 79, 80, 81, 84, 91, 92, 93, 95

L-tryptophan, 141, 162

L-tyrosine, 141, 162

lung cancer, 61, 65, 111, 112, 113, 114, 115, 122

lutein, 64, 65

lycopene, 64–65

lymphoma, 111, 112, 117

lysine, 6, 19

## M

Maalox, 48

macrophages, 18,31, 81, 121

macular degeneration, 65, 66, 71

magnesium, 6, 17, 40, 42, 48, 53, 90–91, 105, 106, 162

magnetic resonance imaging (MRI), 129

manganese, 26, 40, 67–68, 70

marine omega-3 fatty acids, 20, 21, 22,32,35, 37, 86, 145, 146, 156

Massachusetts Institute of Technology, 132

massage, 23, 91, 123

Mavik, 53

Mayeux, Richard, 145

McFarland, J. L., 73, 144, 167

meats
    lean, 43
    as protein source,33
    red meat. See red meat

medications, cautions/concerns with, 24, 46–58, 159. See also specific medications

meditation, 23, 91, 123

melanoma, 72, 111, 115, 116

melatonin, 26, 71–72, 125, 150, 162

melons, 16, 64

memory impairment, 41, 48, 67, 128, 129, 133, 136, 139, 142, 144, 147, 149, 150, 151, 158

memory improvement, 73, 127, 131, 137, 138, 148, 151

memory loss,36, 50, 146

men
    and amount of body fluids, 3
    and cancer, 111
    cholesterol levels in, 80
    and hearing loss, 49
    homocysteine blood serum levels in, 83
    osteoporosis in, 97
    recommended daily intake of B vitamins, 137–139
    recommended daily intake of folic acid, 139
    recommended daily intake of vitamin E, 140

recommended daily protein intake,33

and serotonin, 132

mental activity, 151–152

mental confusion, 137

mental deterioration, 129, 137, 152

mental illness, 137, 138, 139

mental retardation, 138

Mentholatum, 47

mercury, 19, 68

mesothelioma, 115

metabolism, 4, 5, 8, 20, 38–39, 40, 68, 135, 160

Metformin, 54

methionine, 83

methyl salicylate, 47

Mevacor, 50

migraines, 131, 150

milk, 16, 27,33, 63, 66, 67, 99, 100

mineral deficiencies,40–41, 56

minerals, 26,32, 40–43, 66–71, 158 See also acidic minerals; alkaline minerals; essential minerals

Minipress, 53

miscarriages, 24

mitochondria, 8, 25, 68, 70, 116, 124, 142

Mobic, 49

Molecular Endocrinology, 156–157

molybdenum, 40

Monopril, 53

monosaturated fatty acids (omega-9),35

monounsaturated fats, 80

mood impairment, 128

mood improvement, 127, 131, 137–146

mood modulators, 133

mood swings, 129, 130

moods, negative, 7

Motrin, 49

MRI (magnetic resonance imaging), 129

mucilages, 38

mucous, 13, 63, 85

multivatmin pill, 39, 121, 162

Murphy, Brittany, 45
muscle movement, 18
music, listening to, 23, 91, 123
mustard, 65
mutagens, 115
myasthenia gravis, 133
myelin sheath, 135, 139
Mylanta, 48

**N**

Nabumetone, 49
N-acetyl-para-aminopheol (APAP), 46
Naprosyn, 49
nasopharyngeal carcinoma, 116
National Academy of Sciences, 102
National Bone and Joint Disease
    Decade, 98
National Cancer Institute, 38, 122
National Institute of Arthritis and
    Musculoskeletal and Skin Diseases,
    97
National Institutes of Health, 41, 105
National Osteoporosis Foundation, 97
*National Vital Statistics Reports*, 11
natural killer (NK) cells, 6, 18,31, 65,
    121
nectarines, 66
nerve degenerative changes, 138
nerve dysfunction, 139
"nerve food," 133
nervous breakdown, 138
neuritis, 138
neurodegenerative diseases, 59, 60, 72,
    128, 142, 147, 149, 152. *See also*
    *specific diseases*
*Neurology*, 67
neurons, 130–131, 135
Neurontin, 46, 47
neuropathy, 142
neurotransmitters, 21,36, 78, 128, 130–
    134, 135–136, 138, 140, 146, 152
*New England Journal of Medicine*, 50,
    52, 63, 73, 97, 98, 101
*The New York Times*, 54, 101
niacin (B-3), 133, 138

nitrites, 23, 123
nitrosamines, 23, 115
NK (natural killer) cells, 6, 18,31, 65,
    121
nonessential amino acids, 133, 142, 143
non-narcotic analgesics, 49–50
non-steroidal anti-inflammatory drugs
    (NSAIDs), 45, 49
Normodyne, 53
Norvasc, 54
NSAIDs (non-steroidal anti-
    inflammatory drugs), 45, 49
N-telopeptide, 5, 102
numbness, in hands and feet, 138
Nuprin, 49
nutrients
    essential,31, 136, 137–140
    special, for neurostransmitter
        manufacture, 140–144
nutrition
    and acid-alkaline balance, 119
    and cognition, 137
    diet. *See* diet
    eating habits. *See* eating habits
    effect on brain functions, 140, 143,
        152
    as factor in aging, 157
    as factor in heart health, 95,
        157–158
    as factor in osteoporosis, 106, 108
    as factor in reducing risk of age-
        related cancer, 125
    supplements. *See* supplements
nutritional content/value, 20, 42, 122
nutritional deficiencies, 6, 129, 134,
    137
nuts, 16,33, 37, 43, 60, 67, 133
Nytol, 55

**O**

oatmeal, 101, 133
obesity, 3, 22, 73, 79, 121
obsessive-compulsive disorder, 51, 131
*Obstetrics and Gynecology*, 51, 108
oils, 21, 22,35, 44, 60, 162. *See also*

# R

radish, 88, 104, 120
radon gas, 115, 123
Rancho Bernardo Study, 74
rancid fats (lipid peroxides),34–35
*The Real Age Makeover* (Roizen), 63, 74, 168
recipes
    red wine with onion, 94, 163
    for reducing risk of age-related diseases, 162
Reclast, 51, 52
rectum cancer, 111, 112
red meat, 4, 15, 16, 100, 118–119, 158
red peppers, 122
red wine, 93, 94, 147–148, 162, 163
refined grains, 4, 119
refined sugar, 4, 15, 37, 38, 119
Reiter, Russell, 71, 150
resveratrol, 4, 26, 69, 92, 93, 147, 156–157, 162
retinol/retinyl, 63
riboflavin (B-2), 138
rice bran, 100
RNA, 66, 139
Roizen, M. F., 22, 63, 74, 156, 167
Rolaids, 48
Rosai, J., 114

# S

safflower oil, 44
salicylate, 47
saliva, 5, 13. *See also* fasting saliva pH test
salivary glands, 13
salivary lactoperoxidase, 13
salivary lipase, 13
salmon, 7, 19
salt, 158
salt-cured foods, 123
saturated fats
    compared with fully hydrogenated trans fats,34
    effect of, in animals' diets, 145

effect on blood cholesterol level,35, 80
effect on coronary arteries, 85, 86
restriction of, 44, 122
in standard American diet, 20, 28,32, 37
schizophrenia, 72, 131, 132, 139, 143, 150
secretory cells, 13
seeds, 66, 69, 79, 93
selenium, 6, 19, 20, 26, 40, 41, 61, 67, 71
semi-essential amino acids,31,32
senile dementia, 129
senility, 136, 137, 138, 139, 144, 158
series 2 prostaglandins (PGE-2s), 22, 145–146
serotonin, 21, 71, 125, 131–132, 141, 146, 150
serous, 13
Servan-Schreiber, D., 119, 169
sex hormones, 12
sexual dysfunction, 24, 50, 51
sexually transmitted diseases, 121
short-chain omega-3 fatty acids, 21
silicon, 17
simple carbohydrates, 37
single photo emission-computed tomography (SPECT), 129
sirtuin gene, 156–157
sleep, 13, 22, 71, 131, 150, 151
sleep aids/medications, 46, 49, 55–56
sleep deprivation, 151
smoked foods, 123
smoking, 7, 25, 82, 106, 115, 117, 136, 151, 157
snacks,32, 37
SOD (superoxide dismutase), 9, 25, 26, 62, 70–71, 91, 116, 124, 147
sodium, 17, 40, 41, 43, 44, 53
sodium nitrites, 23
sodium phosphate, 107
soft drinks, 14–15, 42, 89, 101, 104, 107, 120
Somiflex, 55

Southwestern Medical Center, 41, 67
soybeans, 133
Spain, cholesterol levels and rates of
  cardiovascular disease in, 84
SPECT (single photo emission-
  computed tomography), 129
sperm counts, 24
spinach, 64, 65, 68, 122
spinal cord, 78
spine, 52, 87, 108
squamous cell carcinoma, 113, 114
squash, 122
standard American diet, 20, 22,32, 100,
  145, 146
statin-type drugs, 27,36, 50, 83, 86, 93.
  *See also specific medications*
*Staying Young* (Oz and Roizen), 22, 156,
  167
steelheads, 7, 19
steroids, 57, 72, 74, 108
stomach cancer, 112, 115, 122
strawberries, 122
stress. *See also* post-traumatic stress
  disorder
    and bone remodeling, 107
    causes of, 22–23
    effect on brain functions, 136, 140
    effect on immunity of, 6, 7, 19,
      117
    hormone (cortisol). *See* cortisol
    and melatonin, 72
    oxidative stress, 60–62, 128, 135,
      146
    reduction/relief, 22–23, 55, 91,
      123, 133, 138, 151, 157
strokes, 22, 27,36, 64, 70, 74, 77, 81,
  82, 84, 85, 93, 113
subclinical malnutrition, 137
sublingual salivary glands, 13
submandibular salivary glands, 13
sugar, 44, 158. *See also* refined sugar
"sugar rush," 37, 38
sulfonylureas, 54
sulfur, 17, 40
sunflower seed oil, 44

Super Poligrip Original, 41
superoxide dismutase (SOD), 9, 25, 26,
  62, 70–71, 91, 116, 124, 147
supplements, 19, 20, 39, 44, 90, 105–
  106, 121, 137, 141, 159, 162 *See also
  specific supplements*
sweet potatoes, 64, 122
Swiss chard, 122
Switzerland, cholesterol levels and rates
  of cardiovascular disease in, 27, 84
synapses, 129, 130, 135, 144, 147
synaptic connectivity, 131
Synthroid, 51, 108

# T

T lymphocytes, 6, 18,31, 66, 121
Tagamet, 48
tai chi, 23, 91, 123
tangerines, 65
tanning devices, 115–116
tardive dyskinesia, 48
tea, 89, 104
Teflon, 23
Tegretol, 51, 108
television, effect of time spent watching,
  18
telomerase, 156
telomeres, 156
Tenormin, 53
testosterone,36
tests
    blood tests, 113
    for cancer, 113
    fasting saliva pH test. *See* fasting
      saliva pH test
    pH tests, 14
Thera-Gesic, 46
thiamin (B-1), 137–138
thiols, 5
thoracic duct, 87
thymus hormones, 12
thyroid hormones, 51, 108
thyroxin, 68
tingling, in hands and feet, 138
tinnitus, 49

tissue fluids, pH levels of, 12, 18
tobacco smoking. *See* smoking
tocopherol (vitamin E), 139–140
Tolinase, 54
tomatoes, 64
Torcetrapib, 27
Toronto General Hospital, 114
toxic chemicals, 16, 23, 24, 46, 56
trace element deficiencies, 40
trace elements, 19,31,32, 40, 121
trachea, 87
trans fats
    and cardiovascular disease, 27, 37,
      90
    described,34–34
    effect of diets rich in, 85
    effect of reducing intake of, 86
    and high omega-6 fatty acid levels,
      27
    in processed foods, 28,32
    restriction of, 44
trauma, 7, 8, 25, 86, 117
trembling, in hands, 138
triglycerides,35, 70, 79, 81, 92, 93
Troglitazone, 55
trout, 7, 19
tryptophan, 6, 19, 71, 125, 132, 141,
    150. *See also* L-tryptophan
Tums, 48
turkey,33, 66
Tylenol, 46, 49
Tylenol PM, 55
type II diabetes, 38, 54, 149
tyrosine, 133. *See also* L-tyrosine

**U**

ultrasound, 113
ultraviolet radiation, 115
United Nations Children's Fund
    (UNICEF), 63
University of California at Berkeley, 149
University of California at San
    Francisco, 156
University of Waterloo, 145
unsaturated fats, 60

unsteadiness, 139
urea,34, 102
urinary incontinence, 139
US Food and Drug Administration
    (FDA), 118

**V**

*Vanity Fair*, 45
Vasolec, 53
vegetables, 5, 16, 20,32,33, 37, 38, 39,
    43, 52, 60, 64, 67, 79, 88, 102, 104,
    120, 122, 141, 147, 153, 162. *See
    also specific vegetables*
villi, 85, 87
vinegar, 15
vinyl chloride, 23, 115, 123
violence, extreme, 131
viral infection, 114, 115, 116, 123
Visken, 53
vitamin A, 6, 19, 25,35, 39, 62–63, 64,
    121, 122
vitamin B, 6, 19, 39, 121, 137
vitamin B-1, 137–138
vitamin B-2, 138
vitamin B-3, 138
vitamin B-5, 138
vitamin B-6, 132, 133, 138
vitamin B-12, 48, 83, 90, 106, 139,
    158
vitamin C, 6, 19, 25, 39, 65–66, 68,
    71, 92, 121, 122, 124
vitamin D, 6, 19,35, 39, 98, 101, 105,
    121
vitamin deficiencies, 40, 56, 137, 140
vitamin E, 6, 19, 25,35, 39, 67, 68, 92,
    121, 124, 137, 139–140
vitamin E (d-alpha-tocopherol), 66,
    139–140
vitamin K, 19,35, 39, 121
vitamins
    antioxidant vitamins, 62–66
    overall, 6,31,32, 38–39, 44, 158
    types of. *See specific vitamins*
    water-soluble, 39
Voltaren, 49

# About the Author

Dr. Liang-Che Tao is professor emeritus of pathology and radiology at the Indiana University School of Medicine, Indianapolis, Indiana. He is also emeritus fellow of the College of American Pathologists, and emeritus fellow of the Royal College of Physicians and Surgeons of Canada.

Before his retirement in 1999, he worked at the Toronto General Hospital and the University of Toronto School of Medicine, Toronto, Ontario, Canada, for twenty-four years. He moved to Indianapolis in 1990 and continued his career at the Indiana University School of Medicine and Indiana University Medical Center as professor of pathology, professor of radiology, and director of the Cytopathology Division.

During those years, he pioneered and fully established the use of image-guided aspiration biopsy and interpretation with specimens from the thorax and abdomen, which he started in 1969 at the Toronto General Hospital. He worked to make deep aspiration biopsy of these sites under the guidance of imaging techniques feasible and practical for clinical use. This combination has become a powerful tool that revolutionized the clinical diagnosis of space-occupying lesions in the thorax and abdomen. What was previously a major diagnostic problem requiring exploratory thoracotomy or laparotomy can now be easily solved by a simple, safe outpatient procedure. Today, the fact that these diagnostic procedures have finally become routine is most certainly due in large part to Dr. Tao's hard work and distinguished career.

He has published five classic text books, including two books on image-guided aspiration biopsy (Tao, L. C. *Guides to Clinical Aspiration Biopsy: Lung, Pleura and Mediastinum.* New York: Igaku-Shoin, 1988. and Tao, L. C. *Transabdominal Fine Needle Aspiration Biopsy.* New York: Igaku-Shoin, 1990.), numerous peer-reviewed research articles, and ten book chapters. His many national and international presentations and workshops, along with his publications, have clearly established him as one of the international leaders in the field of diagnostic cytopathology.

He is also an inventor and holds three US patents: the Tao Brush (for endometrial sampling), the Tao Aspirator (for fine-needle aspiration biopsy), and the Plastic Finger (for safely removing a needle from a syringe).

After his retirement, he shifted his focus to improving his own health, which he noticed to be declining. He reviewed numerous books and research articles on the topic of aging and spent ten years developing theories in the field of aging research. At the same time, he used himself as a guinea pig in trying to improve his health and slow down aging. In so doing, he developed insights into the process of aging and how to help the body regain control over its sovereign territory. Using the "whole-body" approach, Dr. Tao's health problems have diminished to the point where they're almost unnoticeable. Ten years later, he feels younger and more energetic than before. He lives an active life with his wife in the Pacific Northwest.

## Your Record of Morning Fasting Saliva pH Tests

Do this saliva test just after you get out of bed and before you brush your teeth. Fill your mouth with saliva and then swallow it. Do this again and then a third time to ensure that the saliva is clean and contains no bacterial acid products. Put some saliva onto the litmus paper. Or you can use a spoon to hold the saliva, and dip the litmus paper in it. Shake off excess saliva, which may dilute the color. Wait about thirty seconds, and compare the color with the chart.

| Year | Month | Day | pH reading |
|------|-------|-----|------------|
|      |       |     |            |
|      |       |     |            |
|      |       |     |            |
|      |       |     |            |
|      |       |     |            |
|      |       |     |            |
|      |       |     |            |
|      |       |     |            |
|      |       |     |            |
|      |       |     |            |
|      |       |     |            |
|      |       |     |            |
|      |       |     |            |
|      |       |     |            |
|      |       |     |            |
|      |       |     |            |
|      |       |     |            |
|      |       |     |            |
|      |       |     |            |
|      |       |     |            |
|      |       |     |            |
|      |       |     |            |
|      |       |     |            |
|      |       |     |            |
|      |       |     |            |
|      |       |     |            |
|      |       |     |            |
|      |       |     |            |
|      |       |     |            |
|      |       |     |            |
|      |       |     |            |
|      |       |     |            |
|      |       |     |            |

| Year | Month | Day | pH reading |
|------|-------|-----|------------|
|      |       |     |            |
|      |       |     |            |
|      |       |     |            |
|      |       |     |            |
|      |       |     |            |
|      |       |     |            |
|      |       |     |            |
|      |       |     |            |
|      |       |     |            |
|      |       |     |            |
|      |       |     |            |
|      |       |     |            |
|      |       |     |            |
|      |       |     |            |
|      |       |     |            |
|      |       |     |            |
|      |       |     |            |
|      |       |     |            |
|      |       |     |            |
|      |       |     |            |
|      |       |     |            |
|      |       |     |            |
|      |       |     |            |
|      |       |     |            |
|      |       |     |            |
|      |       |     |            |
|      |       |     |            |
|      |       |     |            |
|      |       |     |            |
|      |       |     |            |
|      |       |     |            |
|      |       |     |            |
|      |       |     |            |